APPLYING MOTIVATIONAL THEORY TO HEALTH CARE LEADERSHIP

APPLYING MOTIVATIONAL THEORY TO HEALTH CARE LEADERSHIP

Steven B. Reed, FACHE

Indiana University
Indianapolis

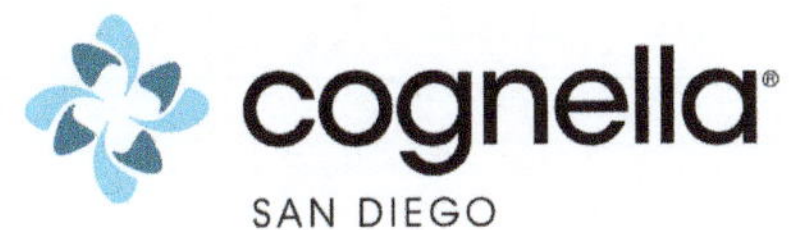

Bassim Hamadeh, CEO and Publisher
Amanda Martin, Executive Publisher
Amy Smith, Associate Editorial Manager
Samantha Hansen, Production Editor
Emely Villavicencio, Senior Graphic Designer
Kylie Bartolome, Licensing Specialist
Natalie Piccotti, Director of Marketing
Kassie Graves, Senior Vice President, Editorial
Alia Bales, Director, Project Editorial and Production

Printed in the United States of America.

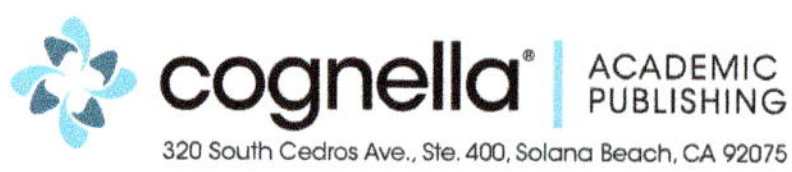

Contents

ACTIVE LEARNING

This book has interactive activities available to complement your reading.

Your instructor may have customized the selection of activities available for your unique course. Please check with your professor to verify whether your class will access this content through the Cognella Active Learning portal (http://active.cognella.com) or through your home learning management system.

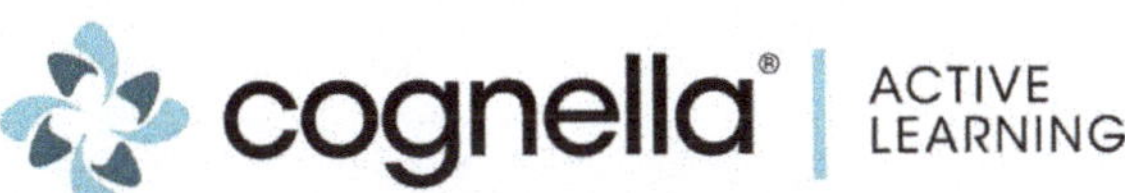

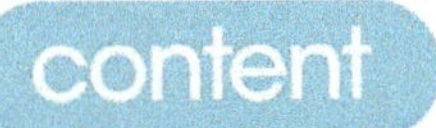

Reviewers

Ellen J. Winiarczyk, EdD
University of Denver, University College, Nonprofit Leadership Master's Program

Dr. Hope Attipoe
Savannah State University

Catherine Rymsha
The University of Massachusetts, Lowell

CHAPTER 1

Introduction

As the world changes, so does health care. The U.S. health care industry has undergone, and will continue to undergo, enormous change in terms of advancements in medical technologies as well our overall knowledge about the human body, disease prevention and diagnosis, diagnostic and therapeutic interventions, clinical capabilities and protocols, and even the environment of care in which health care services are delivered. In addition, our health care system will continue to evolve to meet changes in reimbursement structures, methodologies, and amounts; incentives to promote population health; the supply of health care manpower, supplies, and other critical resources; regulations; accreditation standards, health care reform measures, and more. As the U.S. health care system continues to evolve, it must also meet the evolving needs, wants, and expectations of health care consumers and other stakeholders alike. Today there are growing pressures on health care providers and organizations from virtually all stakeholder segments. Pressures on hospitals include improving access, affordability, safety, quality, and patient experience. This is where leadership—which is about motivating and inspiring others to work hard to achieve organizational goals—is increasingly playing a vital role in health services delivery and with health care delivery systems' ability to meet the evolving needs, wants, and expectations of health care consumers and other stakeholders. Improving the overall performance at all levels of hospitals, health care systems, and health care delivery takes strong, high-performing leadership working closely with a large, diverse workforce that is talented, skilled, highly trained, and experienced—both in clinical and nonclinical aspects. And improving organizational performance takes health care workers who are led and supported by strong leadership that is motivating and inspiring.

Application of Motivational Theories Can Improve Health Care Leadership Effectiveness

Most health care workers go into health care to make an impact—a difference in the lives of other people, the majority of whom they've never seen or met before. Most health care workers are dedicated, caring people who are committed to helping others. For most, working in health care is a calling to service. However, the incredibly dynamic environment, with its increasing demands, challenges, and expectations from all stakeholders, has created a greater need for health care workers to be motivated and inspired to confront the demands and challenges they face and to meet the growing expectations of those they serve. In short, it is more incumbent than ever that health care leaders create a working environment that is motivating and inspiring for their health care workers. Moreover, the practical application of various motivational theories, using techniques and actions highlighted in this handbook, can significantly help a health care leader motivate and inspire their workforce. And when health care workers are motivated and inspired, they are generally more engaged, more caring, more understanding, more productive, and generally perform at a higher level in completing tasks, fulfilling responsibilities, and serving patients.

Health Care Manpower Shortages and Burnout

One of the areas of growing attention and concern for health care workers is burnout. Increasingly, more research is bringing to light the problem of burnout in many health care professions, including with physicians and nurses. This growing body of research is shedding light on the fact that a job and career in health care serving others can take its toll, at some point, given the high and growing demands and challenges placed on health care workers in virtually all lines of work or professions. And while inspiring and motivating leadership, by itself, isn't a panacea for health care worker burnout, it is certainly an aspect that deserves its due consideration given the positive impact it can have. Simply put, motivating and inspiring leadership can make a real difference. Moreover, health care leaders who view their role and responsibility as serving their staffs, which includes motivating and inspiring health care workers who serve hospital patients and families, can make a real difference in helping to stem health care worker burnout, a growing issue in health care today. Besides helping to stem burnout, leadership motivation can help to

- create positive relationships between leaders and staff,
- foster health care worker effort, productivity, and performance,
- create a more pleasant, enjoyable, and caring working environment,
- positively impact employee recruitment and retention,
- improve patient experience and satisfaction, and
- foster problem-solving, performance improvement, and overall financial performance.

The U.S. Health Care System—at a Glance

The U.S. health care system is the largest single employment sector in the world (Laughlin et al., 2021). The U.S. Bureau of Labor Statistics reports there were approximately 21.2 million workers in the U.S. health care industry in 2021 (U.S. Bureau of Labor Statistics, 2022). The National Health Expenditure Accounts (NHEA) estimate that total health care spending in the United States in 2021 was approximately $4.3 trillion, or $12,914 per person. This level of health care spending in 2021 represented 18.3% of the U.S. gross domestic product or GDP (Centers for Medicare & Medicaid Services, 2022). The United States spends more on health care—by far—than any other country in the world. To put this spending in perspective globally, consider this: the $4.3 trillion of annual expenditures on health care in 2021 in the United States surpassed the GDP of every other country in the world except for China and Japan (Centers for Medicare & Medicaid Services, 2022). Does spending $4.3 trillion, or more than 18% of our GDP annually, make the U.S. health care system the best? Not necessarily. From many perspectives the U.S. health care system is one of the greatest in the world. Does the U.S. health care system have opportunities for improvement? Of course, but what other national health care system doesn't have opportunities for improvement? Do all U.S. citizens have equal access to health care services? No, but countries that have a universal health care system don't have equal access either due to some of the same reasons, such as a maldistribution of hospitals and providers; manpower shortages; unavailability of needed drugs, supplies, or other medical resources or technologies in certain areas; long waiting times for common diagnostic and intervention procedures; inadequate funding; and multitiered reimbursement systems and methodologies.

As a country, is the $4.3 trillion or more the United States spends on health care annually too much? That question is frequently debated on a national level, with the implication that our spending on health care is too high; however, what is the right or optimal amount of money that the United States or any other country for that matter should be spending on health care, and exactly what specific criteria should we use to make that determination? Based on universally accepted criteria or determinants used to measure and compare one country's health care system to another, is the United States getting its money's worth? Again, this question is difficult to answer objectively, since many of the factors that contribute to morbidity and mortality—and the other health status indicators commonly used in making an assessment about the performance and effectiveness of a country's health care system—are impacted as much by lifestyles and genetics as the health care system itself. Moreover, the United States is a leading country for lifestyle issues such as alcohol and drug abuse, obesity, stress, lack of physical exercise, and inadequate sleep—just to name a few. The Center for Disease Control (CDC) estimates that approximately half of all premature deaths occurring in the United States are linked to lifestyle. Moreover, indicative of the role that economics and culture can play in health, the CDC found that residents of Alabama, Florida, Georgia, Kentucky, Mississippi, North Carolina, South Carolina, and Tennessee are 28% to 33% more likely to die from a preventable condition than if they lived elsewhere in the United States. Not coincidentally, these states have high smoking and obesity rates, low physical activity rates, and fewer programs for monitoring chronic health conditions (Lubman Rathner, n.d.).

Another important point here is that approximately half of all U.S. health care expenditures are from private monies (vs. governmental programs/funding), including commercial health care insurance companies, private third-party payers, employers, and health care consumers alike, which is far more in terms of total expenditure than any other country in the world. As one of the wealthiest countries in the world, the United States has more public and private health care services available than most other countries, has one of the most robust business and industrial sectors, and overall has one of the most affluent populations as well. Therefore, it stands to reason that as U.S. consumers look for ways to promote their own health and longevity, expenditures on products and services that promote or improve health would be strong.

A Dynamic U.S. Health Care Environment

The environment that hospitals and other health care organizations operate in today is dynamic, with an increasing number of problems, challenges, and opportunities. While there have always been problems, challenges, and opportunities for improvement in the U.S. health care system, it can be argued there are more challenges facing health care leaders today than in any other time in modern U.S. history.

The American College of Healthcare Executives (ACHE) does an annual survey of hospital CEOs on the biggest challenges they face. The survey is confined to CEOs of community hospitals (nonfederal, short-term, nonspecialty hospitals); there were 281 total respondents to the 2023 survey. Here are the top 10 survey results, starting with the most important or biggest challenge they faced in 2023:

1. Workforce challenges (e.g., personnel shortages)
2. Financial challenges
3. Behavioral health/addiction issues
4. Patient safety and quality
5. Governmental mandates
6. Access to care
7. Patient satisfaction
8. Physician–hospital relations
9. Technology
10. Population health management

The average rank given to each issue identified in the ACHE survey was used to place the issue in order of how pressing it is to hospital CEOs. Within each issue listed, respondents identified more specific concerns facing their hospitals. Following are those more specific concerns in order of mention for the number one issue: workforce challenges:

- shortages of registered nurses
- shortages of technicians
- burnout among nonphysician staff

- shortages of therapists
- shortages of physician specialists
- shortages of primary care physicians
- shortages of advanced practice professionals
- managing remote staff
  (ACHE, 2023)

As you look at these two lists, think about the significance and complexities involved in these various challenges in health care. Think more specifically about the challenges pertaining to the workforce, such as personnel shortages and the effect burnout has on staff recruitment, retention, engagement, and motivation. While the number one issue, workforce challenges, clearly is impacted by the motivation of the hospital workforce, isn't the hospital's ability to perform financially, address behavioral health and addiction issues, promote patient safety and quality, and comply with onerous government mandates and the like impacted by the motivation of the hospital workforce as well? Of course! The role that motivation of the workforce plays in all of this is quite significant, and one that health care leaders need to consider as they attempt to address these issues and challenges.

Motivation in the Workplace

Most people will agree that motivation plays a significant role in any workplace environment—even for those who work primarily from home. A work environment that is motivating stimulates us to give greater effort and generally contributes a stronger performance versus a work environment we don't find motivating. A work environment we find motivating helps to tap into our discretionary effort; that is, the amount of effort and performance we are willing to give over and above the minimum job requirements of our position.

When health care managers and workers aren't motivated, effort and performance can suffer. Organizational performance can suffer. Patient care can suffer. The level of motivation of health care managers and workers can impact just about anything and everything in a hospital or health services organization. *Think about it.* The motivation level of health care workers impacts their respective morale, satisfaction, engagement, productivity, creativity, problem-solving, retention, compliance with important procedures and protocols, and their overall effort and performance. In turn, these things directly impact teamwork, collaboration, quality, patient safety, customer service, clinical outcomes—really anything and everything!

Work environments have a long reach, and deep penetration into the psyche of employees. A central part of any organization's working environment is the organizational culture, or how the organization does things. A more formal definition of organizational culture is the values, beliefs, and attitudes of the organizational members. Senior leadership in any organization has the greatest overall influence over the organizational culture. However, organizational culture is best represented by what leadership says, does, supports, recognizes, rewards, promotes, permits, condones, allows, and generally holds employees accountable to. Another way to say this is the organizational culture is best represented by what leadership expresses, manifests, and outwardly demonstrates they believe, value, and want repeated or not repeated.

The Business Case for Leadership Motivation

According to Ken Stella, past hospital administrator and president of the Indiana Hospital Association for over 20 years, "Ongoing leadership motivation in health care is an absolute requirement." This quote came from an interview I conducted with Mr. Stella in 2010.

Here are 10 reasons why health care leaders need to provide motivation to their health care workers on an ongoing basis.

1. Motivated health care workers are more engaged and give more of their best performance.
2. Motivated health care workers are more likely to give more of their discretionary effort.
3. Motivated health care workers are more likely to take responsibility and perform tasks at a higher level.
4. Motivated health care workers are more likely to provide greater customer service and patient experience and satisfaction.
5. Motivated health care workers are more likely to display teamwork and collaborate more effectively with their coworkers and others.
6. Motivated health care workers are more likely to increase their overall productivity.
7. Motivated health care workers are more likely to offer more of their creativity and help problem-solve.

8. Motivated health care workers are more likely to have greater job satisfaction and morale.
9. Motivated health care workers are more likely to help strengthen the overall organizational culture.
10. Motivated health care workers are more likely to stay with the organization, thus improving employee retention.

Common Inner Drives or Motivators

There are countless psychological and related inner drives that motivate health care workers—clinical and nonclinical, management, salaried or rank-and-file hourly employees, and even trustees—to do the work they do. For some, one or two motivating factors may be the overriding, predominant drives for their actions. However, a singular drive or motivating factor, or combination of two or more drives or motivating factors, can be at play at any time, at any moment.

Below you will find an incomplete list of drives or motivating factors. The purpose for highlighting these is to facilitate your own examination and contemplation about what drives or motivates you, colleagues you might work or associate with, or even those you lead or serve in some capacity. Some of these drives or motivating factors listed below are specific, while others are broad, more encompassing, or even more compelling, depending on the circumstances, the respective individual, the environment, the situation at hand, or other related or intervening factors that may be at play at the time:

- pleasant or unpleasant thought
- familiar sound
- familiar smell
- picture that triggers a memory
- desire to achieve a goal or objective
- desire to prove one's ability or value
- pride
- perfectionism
- desire to accomplish a task
- desire to complete assignment or necessary work
- sense of duty
- sense of responsibility, to self or others

- fear of failure
- desire to succeed
- desire to achieve
- desire to serve
- desire to contribute to a cause
- desire to help someone or something
- desire to help make another life better
- pressure to not be fired
- pressure to maintain employment and income
- desire to fulfill a promise or commitment
- an inner passion
- a desire to generate more income

And the list goes on …

The level of motivation that someone experiences can change abruptly or ebb and flow more slowly or deliberately over time. It is common for someone to feel different levels of motivation throughout the course of the day or even work shift with changes in the factors that stimulate internal drives or motivators.

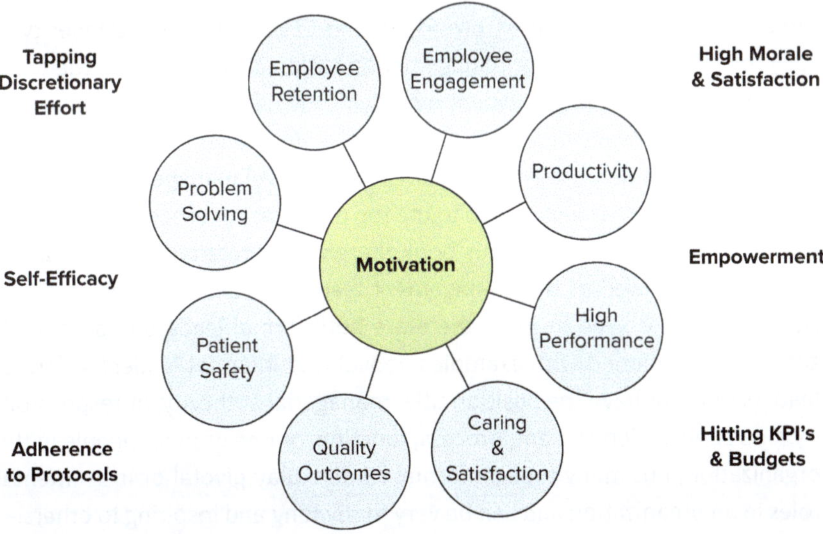

Figure 1.1 Motivation and Its Impact

Management Versus Leadership

In this book, as in practice, the terms management and leadership are used somewhat synonymously and interchangeably; however, management and leadership are technically not the same. Therefore, a few definitions are in order here. The renowned management consultant and author Peter Drucker said that "*management is doing things right; leadership is doing the right things*" (Drucker, 1967, p. 42). Management can be defined as *getting work done through others* while leadership can be defined as *motivating and inspiring others to work hard to achieve organizational goals*. The four basic functions of management include planning, organizing, leading, and controlling. Therefore, leading or leadership is one of the four basic functions of management (Reed, 2018).

In this handbook, a health care leader or health care manager is someone working in a hospital or health service organization who has management authority and responsibility at some level in the organization. Common leadership position titles include team leader, shift leader, charge nurse, nurse manager, unit manager, nurse coordinator, coordinator, supervisor, department manager, director, assistant administrator, vice president, assistant vice president, chief nursing officer, chief operating officer, medical director, chief medical officer, president, and CEO. The word *manager* typically refers to someone in a management position at some level in the organization. The phrase *management team* typically refers to the entire team of managers at all levels in an organization. A *senior leader* refers to someone in a top management, senior level, or executive level management position. The *senior leadership team* refers to the top managers or executive leaders as a unit or group. Throughout this book there will be references to managers and leaders, as well as the management team and senior leadership team. However, please keep in mind there are both formal leaders in an organization (as mentioned with examples above) and informal leaders. Informal leaders may not have the position title, managerial authority, or responsibility for a service, department, process, function, or one or more people in the organization, but many times informal leaders play pivotal or instrumental roles in an organization and can be very motivating and inspiring to others.

As we've already established, a hospital is a labor-intensive organization, with a great number of different, highly specialized positions and workers. There is a high degree of specialization as well as diversity in a typical community hospital. While specialization and diversity have many dimensions, the specialization and diversity of workers vis-à-vis education, knowledge, skills, abilities, and competencies in a typical community hospital are quite impressive. Clinical workers can include primary care physicians, physician specialists, registered nurses, nurse anesthetists, physical therapists, medical lab technologists, radiology technologists, social workers, clinical psychologists, and dieticians. While the vast majority of highly specialized health care workers are clinical, there are other specialized workers that are nonclinical as well.

We frequently think of nonclinical workers in a hospital as support personnel who help facilitate the work performed by workers who are clinical. Nonclinical workers can include plant operations and maintenance workers, biomedical engineers, dosimetrists, patient account representatives, human resource professionals, administrative assistants, and administrators. While it takes a team of interdisciplinary clinical and nonclinical health care workers to provide patient care, it also takes a team of health care leaders with a variety of leadership talents and skills to manage the specialization and diversity of the health care workforce and the operations of a typical community hospital. And it takes health care leaders who can provide strong leadership and motivate and inspire others to successfully lead hospital operations and staff to give their best, and perform at their best, every day.

Many times, when we think of a health care leader providing strong leadership, we think of a senior leader who provides clear and effective vision and strategy, sound budgeting and financial management, or effective recruiting of a diverse team of physicians and other providers to the hospital or health system's provider network. But it truly takes skilled leadership at all levels of a hospital or health service organization to help make the organization's operations and its quality, safety, service and financial performance strong.

Leadership in Health Care

Maybe more than any other time in U.S. history, health care needs effective, high-performing leaders—at all levels of management or leadership. Leadership style is very important, as it impacts employee engagement, employee and organizational accountability, and the ability to bring out the best that each individual health care worker and every health care team has to give. Challenges will only continue to mount for U.S. hospitals and other health care delivery systems and organizations in the future. The operating environment will most certainly become increasingly difficult, and it will take highly effective, high-performing leaders to provide the leadership necessary for hospitals and health service organizations to meet their respective missions, attain their visions, operate efficiently, be financially strong, and provide the highest-quality care and customer service in the safest, most cost-effective manner possible. Strong, effective leadership takes leaders who can motivate and inspire others to give their best every day in the provision of patient care, whether in a direct patient care role or a supportive role.

Leadership Motivation

Leadership provided by a health care manager can be motivating, demotivating, or have no impact on a health care worker's level of motivation. Leadership motivation can involve simple human interactions between health care managers and workers, interpersonal dealings or relationships, or other encounters in the working environment. Leadership motivation can also involve more extensive or involved aspects of the employment relationship, such as completing duties, tasks, and responsibilities, including the process of making and implementing organizational or departmental policies and procedures, training and development opportunities or activities, staffing and work assignments, responses to vacation requests for days off, performance evaluations, matters involving compensation, completion of a project or other assignment involving collaboration and teamwork, or employee recognition or reward. Sometimes it can even be a health care manager's reaction to a worker's idea or suggestion that can be motivating or demotivating. In essence, almost everything a health care manager does or says can impact a worker's level of motivation in some way.

In today's challenging health care environment, it takes health care workers who are committed, engaged and motivated to render great patient experience in a friendly and safe environment, with quality outcomes, in an efficient and effective manner that helps the organization fulfill its mission and create overall strong hospital performance. Again, all of this takes leaders who can motivate and inspire health care workers to be their best and give their best.

As used in this book, the phrase *leadership motivation* relates to a health care manager's actions and behaviors that are designed or intended to motivate health care workers, and the impact or effect of those actions or behaviors on motivation. The assumption is that leadership motivation is something intentional that a health care manager says or does in an attempt to motivate others. However, a health care manager can be motivating without really being aware of it, or without having the intent or making a conscience effort to be motivating. By the same token, a health care manager can be demotivating without really knowing it. We can assume that most health care managers never intend to be demotivating; however, it happens.

A health care leader can't give an employee motivation; motivation is something that lies within each of us, and is different for each of us. What a leader can do is connect with or stimulate the inner drives that motivate an employee. The vast majority of health care workers and caregivers share one or more drives or motivators around caring and service, and work in health care to serve and make a difference for others. Therefore, while there are different drives that motivate each of us, the majority of health care workers and caregivers have a desire—and many a passion—to serve and make a positive difference in the lives of others. This passion is a common denominator among the vast majority of health care workers and caregivers, and a key for health care leaders looking to motivate health care employees.

Health care is a business of health care workers caring for others, serving others, and making a difference for others. Health care is about people caring for people and giving of themselves to others—their gifts, talents, and abilities—in the provision caring and compassionate service. Now, you might be thinking, *but aren't you just talking about physicians, nurses, and other direct patient caregivers*? No. Of course this discussion includes direct patient caregivers, but it also includes indirect patient caregivers. This discussion includes employees that work in the hospital cafeteria, biomedical engineering, environmental services, patient accounts, and administration. It also includes epidemiologists, nurses, statisticians, and other workers in county and state health departments; patient account representatives and claims processors working for third-party administrators or health insurance payers; and myriad of other health care workers in a variety of health services organizations and agencies. And as a general rule, health care workers in any segment of health care perform better when they are motivated to do so.

Therefore, as stated by Ken Stella,

> "Ongoing leadership motivation in health care is an absolute requirement."
>
> (Ken Stella, personal communication)

Motivation is a necessity for caregivers working in direct patient care, health care employees performing a supportive role or function that supports direct patient caregivers, and health care managers and leaders responsible for managing the operations of a health services organization. And in today's dynamic and demanding health care working environment, it takes leadership that is motivating and inspiring for health service organizations and health care workers and caregivers alike to excel—by being at their best and giving their best.

Health Care Leaders Can Find Motivation Through Management by Walking Around

Can a health care leader who isn't motivated and inspired by the purpose of the work they do motivate and inspire others? Probably not, as it is hard to imagine an unmotivated health care leader being able to motivate others effectively. How do health care leaders motivate and inspire themselves? While the answer to this question is probably different for each leader, here is something I would like to share from my own experience.

As a hospital administrator, I found most experiences when I was out and about in the hospital—walking around or making administrative rounds—to be motivating and inspiring. Seeing, acknowledging, recognizing, and interacting with physicians, direct patient caregivers, and supportive caregivers such as general service workers, and observing them doing great work, was always inspiring. Moreover, it was always enjoyable and rewarding getting to know employees on a more personal level; learning who they are as a person; learning a little about their families, their personal stories, and their goals for the work they do every day; and seeing and hearing about the important contributions they make for their coworkers, colleagues, patients, families, and the organization as a whole. It can make a difference when a health care leader gets to know the people of the organization and sees the good work they do up close: it engenders a greater sense of understanding, respect, appreciation, and even gratitude for them.

Moreover, the importance of health care leaders having presence and visibility with frontline health care workers where the care is being delivered and work is being done cannot be overstated. Health care workers want to see leaders out in the organization, and leadership visibility can provide tangible proof that a leader cares about the health care workers, the patients, the care being delivered, and the work being done. While this point is true for all health care leaders, it is especially true for senior leaders. For some health care workers, it is this type of leadership visibility, along with leadership interaction with employees, on which they base their perception about whether senior leaders care about their employees and the work they do. But there is more to this story—much more!

The work of most hospital administrators, especially those in senior executive leadership positions, involves writing and reviewing reports, budgets, financial statements, plans, emails, memos, letters, policies and procedures, contracts, and other documents. Senior leaders are involved in a lot of decisions, and a lot of meetings as well. Sometimes it is easy for a senior leader to lose sight—even become a bit disconnected from—care delivery that is happening every day. For a senior leader to stay connected or reconnect to the heart of why the organization exists, and why the senior leader got into health care in the first place—to serve patients and make a difference in their lives—can be one of the most motivating and inspiring things they, or any health care leader for that matter, can do. And maybe the quickest and most effective way a health care leader can stay connected or reconnect to the mission of serving others and making a difference for patients is through management by walking around (MBWA). MBWA is about a leader physically going out in the organization and observing patient care being delivered and supportive work being provided firsthand, and seeing how it is making a positive difference in countless lives and for the organization as a whole.

The vast majority of health care workers are well-trained, caring, and compassionate professionals who give their best every day in the service of others, provide them with the best quality of care and customer service possible, and make a real difference. To see this type of caring service, supportive work, and professional behavior towards patients is inspiring and motivating—with almost every patient a virtual, and sometimes actual, stranger to their caregivers. The passion for serving others is virtually ubiquitous in health care, and it is truly a calling; a calling to make a difference; a calling to live a life that makes an impact. And any time a person connects or reconnects to their passion, they become inspired, as it brings them purpose and fulfillment.

Motivators and Zappers

As a senior lecturer at Indiana University, I teach a course in the Master of Health Administration program with graduate students in their last semester, referred to as the capstone course. One of the activities I do in the classroom with students is have them compile a list of things that leaders do that motivate them ("motivators") and a list of things that leaders do that demotivate them ("zappers"). We compile and discuss these two lists in class, then post the list online to the course's learning management system for the students' reference and use. Facilitating this exercise in the classroom is always fun and interesting, and it helps get students thinking about what things leaders do that they find both motivating and demotivating, and what they might want to incorporate into their own leadership style. The following list consists of 20 motivators and 20 zappers that have been generated by students from the past several years of teaching this course. As you review these two lists, ask yourself these questions as they relate to your own experience:

1. Which items on each list do you agree with?
2. Which items on each list do you disagree with?
3. Based on your own experience, what items would you add to each list?
4. Which items on each list are your biggest "pet peeves" or would you rate as most significant?
5. Which item(s) from the list of motivators could you enhance, foster to a greater extent, or incorporate into your own leadership style?
6. What action steps should you take to enhance, foster, or incorporate one or more motivators into your own leadership style?
7. Which item(s) from the list of zappers should you be more cognizant of not doing/avoiding in your leadership style?
8. What action steps should you take to not do or avoid one or more zappers from showing up in your leadership style?

9. Is it possible that one or more of the zappers is something you do, or could do, without even realizing it (a blind spot, if you will)?
10. Do you have a trusted mentor or someone who could provide you with *outside insight* to help you better determine if you might have a blind spot about one or more of the items on the zappers list?

Motivators

- Having/being provided autonomy
- Short-term successes
- Encouragement
- Affirmation
- When a leader believes in me
- Remembering the "why" (I am doing the work)
    - Connect to the patient and the bigger picture
- Investing in professional growth/development
- Trusting the team (having mutual trust)
- Taking the initiative and just do it: don't wait or over-analyze
- Being acknowledged/recognized
- A leader who admits a mistake
- A positive organizational culture
- Intangible/tangible rewards and incentives
- Empowering others on the team—encouraging and helping them with their work
- Keeping employees informed of where we are going and how we are going to get there
- Setting attainable goals with high success probability and "feeling the wins" no matter what size
- Publicly recognizing high achievers
- Participatory leadership
- Creating the opportunity and delegating—ensuring that opportunities are given out

Zappers

- Lack of mutual trust
- Unclear expectations followed by criticism
- Being micromanaged

- Someone who speaks poorly of others
- Someone who thinks they are always "right" (and they aren't)
- Talks more than they listen
- Doesn't understand or appreciate a person's work or effort
- Poorly performing managers/leaders
- Being tasked with overly basic/simple tasks
- Lack of communication and transparency
- Overworking—too many tasks, forced overtime work, etc.
- Tolerating poor performance of others
- A pessimistic leader
- Derailing momentum secondary to red tape, unnecessary approvals, etc.
- Leading by example in a negative way
- Lack of accountability
- Lack of honesty
- Not having a why or reason for why something that someone is doing is important
- Having meetings that could have been emails
- Boss acting too important, too busy to care, and not respecting the employee's time or personal life

MOTIVATIONAL QUOTES

Quotes can be motivating. Here are fifteen quotes that I hope you find motivating.

> "What a man can be, he must be. This need we call self-actualization."
>
> Abraham Maslow (Maslow, n.d.)
>
> "If you plan on being anything less than you are capable of being, you will probably be unhappy all the days of your life."
>
> Abraham Maslow (Maslow, 1971).
>
> "A failure is not always a mistake; it may simply be the best one can do under the circumstance. The real mistake is to stop trying."
>
> B. F. Skinner (Skinner, 1971)

"It's the job of a manager not to light the fire of motivation, but to create an environment to let each person's personal spark of motivation blaze."

Frederick Herzberg (Segal, 2003, p. 12)

"The best way to predict the future is to create it."

Peter Drucker (Drucker, 1986)

"If you want something new, you have to stop doing something old."

Peter Drucker (Drucker, 2013)

"The quality of leadership, more than any other single factor, determines the success or failure of an organization."

Fred E. Fiedler (Fiedler & Chemers, 1974)

"You can become an even more excellent person by constantly setting higher and higher standards for yourself and then by doing everything possible to live up to those standards."

Brian Tracy (Tracy, 2020)

"We are what we repeatedly do. Excellence, then, is not an act, but a habit."

Aristotle (Durant, 1926)

"The only person you are destined to become is the person you decide to be."

Ralph Waldo Emerson (Daily Reflections, 2023)

"Be miserable. Or motivate yourself. Whatever has to be done, it's always a choice."

Wayne Dyer (Dyer, 2010)

"When you dance, your purpose is not to get to a certain place on the floor. It's to enjoy each step along the way."

Wayne Dyer (Dyer, 2011)

> "The greater danger for most of us lies not in setting our aim too high and falling short, but in setting our aim too low and achieving our mark."
>
> Michelangelo (Quotes of Michelangelo, 2011)

History Versus the Past

Just a quick note about history and the past. The past is all time that has come before us. History is what we have chosen to record, document, and/or remember about the past; therefore, history is a subset of the past, and one that is not perfect, but incomplete—by definition. However, we can learn from the past, as well as our own personal and professional history or experience, which many argue may be the best teacher of all. Moreover, some will argue that history always tends to repeat itself, so history or experience may very well be the best teacher of all, as it is somewhat reoccurring. One interesting thing about learning through our experiences is that we typically don't learn the lesson until after we've had the experience. This handbook provides learning and guidance on motivational theories and their application in health care leadership based upon history, personal and professional experience, and lessons learned from multiple sources and people.

Motivational Theories Explored in This Handbook

This handbook will attempt to help you learn as well as gain a deeper understanding about motivational theory and how to apply it as a health care leader. We will examine a number of motivational theories that have been promulgated throughout history based upon experiments, empirical evidence, research, and other writings. The motivational theories explored in this handbook are largely based on the experience and wisdom of renowned psychologists, researchers, theorists, and health care leaders who were active learners with a healthy sense of curiosity. This handbook is designed to help you—whether a student attending a college or university, or a student of leadership working in the field of health care management looking for additional ideas, strategies, action steps, and overall guidance—more effectively motivate health care workers.

The motivational theories highlighted in this handbook are based on past research-based discoveries, empirical evidence, hypotheses, ways of thinking, and theories that have been promulgated through various writings and interpretations over time. This handbook does not address nor attempt to cover all the motivational theories that have been discovered or promulgated and are available in today's literature. Moreover, there are a number of motivational theories that have evolved directly from those covered in this handbook, or expanded upon ways of thinking about a respective motivational theory covered in this handbook, that won't be mentioned. This handbook does not highlight, address, nor attempt to cover the various categories that have been used to organize motivational theories, such as content theories, process theories, effectance theories, reversal theories, learned helplessness theories, or other categories. This handbook does, however, reference scientific management and several theories which attempt to analyze and synthesize workflows and improve efficiency and productivity The motivational theories featured and examined in this handbook all have relevance for health care leadership, leadership motivation, and health care workers. The actual application of the featured motivational theories specifically in health care leadership is based upon methods and techniques highlighted in the available literature, as well as the experience of this author and several other hospital and health care leaders this author has known, worked with, and/or personally interviewed. One point of caution here: what motivates one person, and what motivational theory may be best to apply for that one person, may not work or be the best for someone else.

Motivation and motivational theories work differently for different people: one size does not fit all.

Theory Versus Practice

There is a well-known adage: *"In theory, theory and practice are the same. In practice, they aren't."* It stands to reason that many times there is a gap between theory and practice. Why? For one thing, there are many variables in practice that aren't part of the corresponding theory. Another reason may be that theories don't apply themselves, and typically it takes the skills and abilities of a practitioner to apply a theory correctly, appropriately, or effectively.

In most every case, the skills of a theoretician are not the same as the skills of a practitioner, as one must be able to translate the knowledge into action in real practice.

What is the difference between theory and practice? Theory is "a supposition or a system of ideas intended to explain something, especially one based on general principles independent of the thing to be explained;" "a set of principles on which the practice or an activity is based;" or "an idea used to account for a situation or justify a course of action" (New Oxford American Dictionary, n.d.). Practice, on the other hand, is "the actual application or use of an idea, belief, or method, as opposed to theories relating to it." Practice is "the customary, habitual, or expected procedure or way of doing of something," such as current nursing practice (Oxford Languages, n.d.).

In my personal experience, the motivational theories presented and explored in this handbook are those that can be successfully applied in practice to varying degrees by most any hospital or health care manager or leader. In other words, the motivational theories promulgated in this handbook are practical, relevant, and effective when appropriately applied by hospital and health care managers and leaders in practice. Moreover, for a hospital or health care manager to be as effective as possible, they must have the requisite knowledge, understanding, skills, and abilities to apply the various motivational theories promulgated in this handbook in practice.

Motivational Theories Explored in This Handbook

Motivation has played an integral part in the human condition since, well, humans have been alive on earth. Suffice it to say that's been a long time; however, it wasn't until instinct theory was promulgated in the late 19th and early 20th century that motivational theory began to emerge.

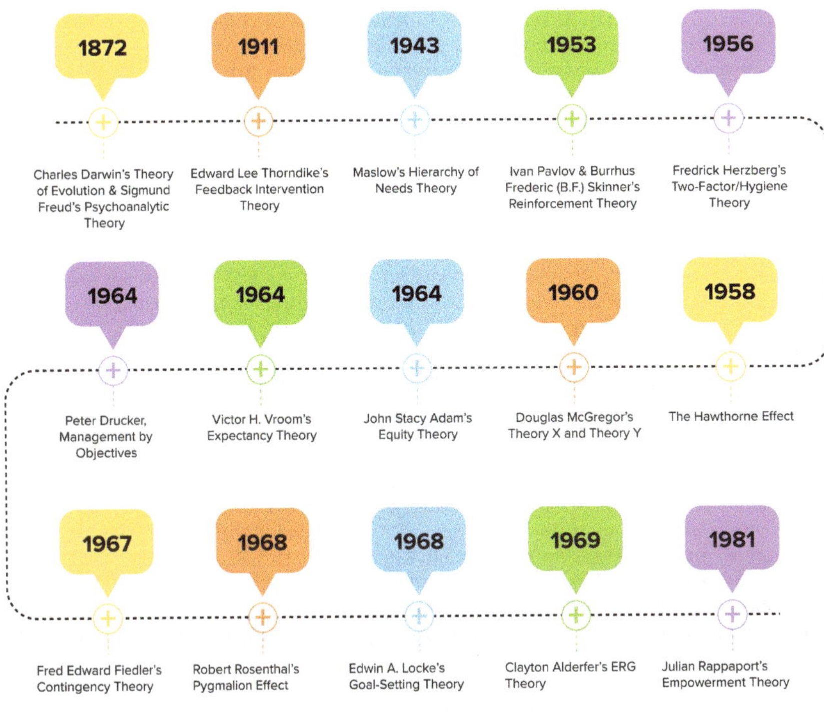

Figure 1.2 Timeline

References

American College of Healthcare Executives. (February 13, 2023). *Survey: Workforce challenges cited by CEOs as top issue confronting hospitals in 2022* [Press release]. https://www.ache.org/about-ache/news-and-awards/news-releases/survey-workforce-challenges-cited-by-ceos-as-top-issue-confronting-hospitals-in-2022

Centers for Medicare & Medicaid Services. (2022, December 14). *National health spending grew slightly in 2021* [Press release]. https://www.cms.gov/newsroom/press-releases/national-health-spending-grew-slightly-2021

Daily Reflections. (2023, March 16). "The only person you are destined to become is the person you decide to be."-Ralph Waldo Emerson. Medium; Medium. https://medium.com/@officialprpatel002/the-only-person-you-are-destined-to-become-is-the-person-you-decide-to-be-ralph-waldo-emerson-13280dfc2e1d#:~:text=Medium-

Drucker, P. F. (1967). *The effective executive.* Harper & Row.

Drucker, P. F. (1986). *The leader of the future.* Jossey-Bass Publishers.

Drucker, P. F. (2013). *People and performance.* Routledge.

Durant, W. (1926). *The story of philosophy: The lives and opinions of the world's greatest philosophers.* Simon & Schuster.

Dyer, W. W. (2010, July 12). Be miserable. Or motivate yourself. Whatever has to be done, it's always your choice [Facebook post]. https://www.facebook.com/drwaynedyer/posts/be-miserable-or-motivate-yourself-whatever-has-to-be-done-its-always-your-choice/131747816860355/

Dyer, W. W. (2011, October 5). When you dance, your purpose is not to get to a certain place on the floor. It's to enjoy each step along the way [Facebook post]. https://www.facebook.com/drwaynedyer/posts/when-you-dance-your-purpose-is-not-to-get-to-a-certain-place-on-the-floor-its-to/10150345211771030/

Fiedler, F. E., & Chemers, M. M. (1974). *Improving leadership effectiveness: The leader match concept.* John Wiley & Sons.

Laughlin, L., Anderson, A., Martinez, A., & Gayfield, A. (2021, April 5). Who are our health care workers? U.S. Census Bureau. https://www.census.gov/library/stories/2021/04/who-are-our-health-care-workers.html

Lubman Rathner, J. (n.d.). CDC: Nearly half of U.S. deaths can be prevented. Laborers' Health & Safety Fund of North America. https://www.lhsfna.org/cdc-nearly-half-of-u-s-deaths-can-be-prevented/

Maslow, A. H. (1971). The Farther Reaches of Human Nature. Penguin Publishing Group.

Maslow, A. H. (n.d.). What a man can be, he must be. This need we call self-actualization. https://psychclassics.yorku.ca/Maslow/motivation.htm

New Oxford American Dictionary. (n.d.). *Theory*. New Oxford American Dictionary (3 Ed.). https://www.oxfordreference.com/display/10.1093/acref/9780195392883.001.0001/m_en_us1298203?rskey=HY3Flq&result=85909

Oxford Languages. (n.d.). *Practice*. In Oxford Languages. https://www.oed.com/dictionary/practice_n?tab=factsheet#28709773

Quotes of Michelangelo. (2011). Henri Matisse. https://www.michelangelo.org/michelangelo-quotes.jsp

Segal, M. (2003). *Quick guide to the four temperaments and creativity.* Telos Publications.

Skinner, B. F. (1971). *Beyond freedom and dignity.* Hackett Publishing Company.

Tracy, B. [@BrianTracy]. (2020, May 13). You can become an even more excellent person by constantly setting higher and higher standards for yourself and then by doing everything. [Post]. X. https://x.com/BrianTracy/status/1259138325501415424

U. S. Bureau of Labor Statistics. (2022, March 7). Over 16 million women worked in health care and social assistance in 2021. *The Economics Daily.* https://www.bls.gov/opub/ted/2022/over-16-million-women-worked-in-health-care-and-social-assistance-in-2021.htm

Creditlines

Fig. 1.2: Copyright © 2014 Depositphotos/ankudi.

CHAPTER 2

Charles Darwin and Sigmund Freud's Instinct Theory of Motivation

Have you ever had an experience when something was telling you—something inside of you, call it instincts, gut feel, or intuition—about another person, problem, situation, solution, language, action, behavior, or even danger in your immediate surroundings? Have you ever had a feeling about something you couldn't explain, but you knew that feeling was accurate or at least something you should pay attention to or follow? Did you follow your instincts or intuition? Were you correct in doing so? How often do you follow your instincts or intuition, and what are the typical signs you look for when doing so?

A classic example of following one's instincts or intuition in health care is when a physician or nurse goes in to examine a patient in a hospital bed and the physician or nurse quickly realizes there is something wrong with the patient but doesn't exactly know what. The physician or nurse heeds or listens to their instincts or intuition and takes action to have the patient tested with diagnostic imaging, blood work, or other means and discovers there really was something else going on with the patient. It wasn't the physician's or nurse's clinical skills per se that came into play at the time—it was their instincts or intuition. All of us are born with instincts and intuition, and many of our basic instincts are the same or at least very similar; however, how we use or apply those instincts or intuition can be very different.

Background and Overview

Charles Darwin was a British naturalist who proposed the theory of biological evolution by natural selection. Darwin defined evolution as "descent with modification," an idea that species change over time, give rise to new species, and share a common ancestor.

Darwin's theory of evolution was first promulgated in his book *On the Origin of Species*, published in 1859. In his book, Darwin described how organisms evolve over generations through the inheritance of physical or behavioral traits. While different organisms have variations in traits, it is the individual traits best suited for the environment that enable species to survive and evolve, and the offspring to inherit those traits. Over time it is the traits that allow the species to adapt, survive, and reproduce that will manifest through genetics (although Darwin didn't know about genetics at that time, or the role of genetics at the level of DNA as a mechanism for traits to be passed on from one generation to the next).

Sigmund Freud was born in 1856 in what is today Czechia. Freud was a physiologist, physician, and psychologist who introduced personality theory, stating that everyone has an id, their primal instincts, a superego that contains a sense of morality, and an ego that balances the two. Freud's most significant contribution to science might be his theory of how the mind works with his discovery of a method of helping people in mental distress called psychoanalysis, which is still used extensively today in the field of behavioral health.

In his first theory, Freud suggested that all humans have the same (or similar) motivations due to our similar biological programming, and that the basis of all motivations is survival. Those motivations are social instincts, security instincts, reproductive instincts, and basic instincts of life, which create self—also called the ego instincts.

Later, Freud modified his theory to suggest there were two primary types of instincts: (a) life drive, which deals with self-preservation (to quench one's thirst or hunger, or to avoid pain) and reproduction, and (b) death instincts, or a natural desire to "re-establish a state of things that was disturbed by the emergency of life." Freud believed that life instincts largely tempered the desire for death (Freud, 1920, as cited in Cherry, 2023).

While both Darwin and Freud's instinct theories have similarities, there are certainly differences as well. Nevertheless, in general, instinct theory may be summarized as drives, urges, impulses, tensions, pressures, or motivations which are innate to all human beings, but do not necessarily drive or manifest themselves to the same degree or in the same way for each of us. The ego—which shapes and drives how a person perceives themselves—may play a major role in how an individual goes about prioritizing and pursuing their instinctive motivations (de Lauretis, 2008; Freud, 1933).

Instinct Theory and Emotional Intelligence

Interestingly, instinct theory may be the original body of thinking and knowledge about self-awareness, self-assessment, self-understanding, and the insight a person has about how they show up in the world, interact with individuals and groups, and are perceived by others. Instinct theory would suggest this self-awareness is based on a person's natural instincts. Today, there is much emphasis placed on the important role emotional intelligence plays in leadership. The current body of knowledge and thinking about emotional intelligence (EI) and its critical role and importance in leadership is well documented and promulgated in a plethora of journals and books, as well as other mediums of dissemination, teaching, and learning. Instinct theory has some similarities to EI.

A health care leader's instincts will impact their decision-making. Moreover, when a health care leader interacts with a health care worker, she will do so—at least in part—using her own instincts and experiences. Moreover, much of her own instincts will be formed through her experiences in life and in leadership, in conjunction with her own personality or how she is hardwired (through genetics).

Most high-performing leaders learn how to use their instincts in order to effectively make decisions; to interact with, collaborate with, and understand others; and to be positively perceived and effectively understood by others. Moreover, in a hospital or other health service setting, it may be even more important for the leader to be in control and in tune with her instincts, and display a positive and likeable persona, as well as to model the way for others, exhibiting positive and effective instincts and EI in an empathetic, caring, and compassionate manner. Many health care workers will take their cues or understanding about what is important and how to behave from the example set by their immediate supervisor, as well as other health care leaders in an organization. One overall conclusion that can be drawn about instinct theory and its impact on employees is this:

> The instincts of a health care leader help shape and govern how they interact with people.

How a health care leader interacts with employees will impact how employees feel about the leader as well as their overall employment relationship. How employees feel about their leader and their overall employment relationship impacts their level of engagement. How a health care leader performs in this regard serves as a model or example for employees to follow. In turn, the level of employee engagement and how employees use their own instincts to interact with others in a hospital or health service organization environment significantly impacts their coworkers, colleagues, boss, and other health care managers—not to mention the patients and families they serve. Therefore:

> Health care leaders should be aware of the role their instincts play in their everyday interactions with employees and others—both individually and in groups—and how their behavior in this regard is modeling the way for others.

Heightening a health care leader's own self-awareness, understanding, and insight about the role their instincts play in their everyday interactions with others, as well as decision-making, will take thoughtful self-reflection on their part. Many instincts that help drive or control a health care leader's decisions and interactions with others may reside in their own subconscious, which can only be tapped into and understood through thoughtful self-reflection.

Key Takeaways for Health Care Leaders

Health care workers have the same drives and motivations as the rest of humanity, which is to say those drives are instinctive or innate to the human species. However, those instincts or motivations don't manifest the same way in everyone, and an individual's personality or ego is a factor that shapes and molds how their instincts are prioritized or manifested. Therefore, health care managers need to know and understand each subordinate on a personal level in order to know and understand how their basic life instincts (social, security, reproductive, and ego instincts) drive or motivate them in everyday life and in a work environment.

Health care managers also need to be aware of their own basic life instincts and how these drive or motivate them in everyday life, in a work environment, and in their own leadership style. What impact does a health care manager's ego (or innate personality) have on their pursuit of satisfying their own life instincts on a regular, routine basis, and how does this manifest in their leadership style with others?

LEADERSHIP ACTION STEPS FOR THE INSTINCT THEORY OF MOTIVATION

1. Health care managers need to be aware at all times of their own basic life instincts and how these drive or motivate them in everyday life, in a work environment, and in their own leadership style.
2. Health care managers need to be aware at all times of their ego (or innate personality) and how their personality molds, shapes, and directs their thoughts and actions in pursuit of satisfying their own life instincts on a regular, routine basis. Moreover, health care managers need to be aware at all times of their own personality and how their innate or natural tendencies or drives manifest in their own leadership style with their subordinates and others.
3. Health care managers should be cognizant of their intuition regarding people, problems, situations, solutions, language, behaviors—even their immediate surroundings. When a health care manager allows him/herself to use his/her instincts can be valuable in assessing or evaluating people, problems, solutions, language, actions, behaviors—even their immediate surroundings.
4. Health care managers should get to know their subordinates (as well as coworkers and colleagues) on a personal level in order to know and understand how their basic life instincts (social, security, reproductive, and ego instincts) drive or motivate them in everyday life including in a work environment. This understanding of life instincts with subordinate's and others will provide health care managers with insight into how they might shape and mold their own leadership style to be most effective.

5. Health care managers should provide a physical working environment and culture for subordinates that positively appeals to their instincts and promotes a positive social working environment that is safe, secure, and appeals to individual's as well as the team's collective personality.

Assessing One's Leadership Style and Instinct Theory

The following questions are designed to prompt reflection and self-assessment, and to promote better understanding and insight about how you—as a student, health care manager, or leader—can use or are using instinct theory with your own leadership style. Use the following 5-point Likert scale for this assessment:

5 = Always 4 = Sometimes 3 = Neutral 2 = Seldom 1 = Rarely/Never

1. I am routinely and consistently self-aware and cognizant of my own basic life instincts and how these drive or motivate me in everyday life, in a working environment, and in my own leadership style, and look for signs and clues to heighten my self-awareness ongoing.

   5 4 3 2 1

2. I know and understand my personality characteristics, drivers, and motivators. I am routinely and consistently self-aware and cognizant of my own ego (or innate personality) and how my personality molds, shapes, and directs my own thoughts and actions in pursuit of satisfying my own life instincts, and in my own leadership style with subordinates and others.

   5 4 3 2 1

- List two or three of the most frequent ways your personality characteristics impact your thoughts and actions as a leader:
    A.
    B.
    C.

3. I am self-aware and cognizant of my own instincts and frequently use my intuition in assessing or evaluating people, problems, situations, solutions, language, behaviors—even the safety and security in my surroundings.

   5 4 3 2 1

4. I get to know and understand my subordinates (as well as coworkers and colleagues) on a personal level ongoing in order to know and understand how their basic life instincts (social, security, reproductive, and ego instincts) drive or motivate them in everyday life, including in a working environment.

   5 4 3 2 1

5. I work to provide a physical working environment and culture for subordinates that positively appeals to their instincts and promotes a positive social working environment and culture that is safe, secure, and appeals to individual's as well as the team's collective personality.

   5 4 3 2 1

____

____

____

____

References

Cherry, K. (2024, April 22). Freud's Concepts of Thanatos and Eros: Understanding the life (Eros) and death (Thanatos) drives. Verywell Mind. https://www.verywellmind.com/life-and-death-instincts-2795847

Darwin, C. (1859). *On the origin of species by means of natural selection, or the preservation of favoured races in the struggle for life.* John Murray.

de Lauretis, T. (2008). Basic instincts: An illustrated guide to Freud's theory of drives. In T. de Lauretis (Ed.), *Freud's drive: Psychoanalysis, literature and film* (pp. 15–33). Palgrave Macmillan.

Freud, S. (1933). *New introductory lectures on psycho-analysis* (W. J. H. Sprott, Trans.). W. W. Norton & Company.

CHAPTER 3

Edward Lee Thorndike's Feedback Intervention Theory

One question that most health care workers have is, *How does my supervisor think that I am doing*? Students have this same question regarding the work they do in the classroom: *How does my teacher think that I am doing*? At most competitive sporting events there is some type of scoreboard so the players—and the fans—know how the players and the teams are doing. A scoreboard acts as a vehicle to provide immediate and ongoing feedback. Feedback on performance is needed in health care—just as it is on the playing field. Feedback is critical to understanding how one is performing, and where changes in effort or performance might be needed to achieve the desired goal or objectives. Feedback is a central component of the basic management function of controlling: monitoring progress towards goal achievement and taking corrective action as needed (Reed, 2018).

Background and Overview

In the beginning of the 19th century, scholars were interested in how to predict individual behavior and what factors influenced performance change. Researchers were focused initially on simple variable analyses, but later began to evaluate feedback that influenced individual performance and behavior. In 1898, Edward Lee Thorndike began investigating how animals learn. Subsequently, Thorndike began investigating feedback intervention using animals, then later humans, as test subjects. Thorndike believed that behavior is predictable and stated: "Of several responses made to the same situation, those which are accompanied or closely followed by satisfaction to the animal will, other things being equal, be more firmly connected with the situation, so that, when it recurs, they will be more likely to recur; those which are accompanied or closely followed by discomfort to the animal will, other things being equal, have their connections with that situation weakened, so that, when it recurs, they will be less likely to occur. The greater the satisfaction or discomfort, the greater the strengthening or weakening of the bond." (Thorndike, 1911, p. 244). In other words, positive feedback was equated with positive reinforcement and negative feedback with negative reinforcement. Moreover, positive and negative reinforcement assist both learning and performance. Thorndike called this initial feedback intervention research the *law of effect* (Olencevicius, 2019).

In developing the *law of effect* Thorndike performed an experiment with cats, which were placed in a specially designed experiment cage called a "puzzlebox." The door of the cage was locked by a simple latch. Outside the cage, Thorndike placed a piece of salmon. The cat was placed in the box and could freely move about the inside. It could see and smell the fish but couldn't reach it from the cage. After some time, the cat began maneuvers by extending its paws through the bars to reach the fish, but without success. After a few unsuccessful attempts, the cat started scratching at the bars of the cage and rushed around inside. Accidentally it hit the latch on the door and the door was opened. The cat went out and ate the fish. The total escape reaction time was measured. The cat was placed back into the cage and a new piece of fish was served again. The cat repeated the process and by hitting the latch one more time went out and successfully reached the fish. This process was repeated multiple times. Thorndike noticed that by repeating this experiment, less time was spent opening the door and the releasing of the latch became faster. Gradually the cat stopped extending its paws through the bars and focused its activities on the latch. Later, it moved immediately to trying to open the door by hitting the latch. After some time, the cat developed an efficient and fast way to open the door. Later, experiments with more complicated door opening schemes were performed, where a few locking mechanisms were involved (Cherry, 2023).

Such changes of cat behavior incorporate learning (Olencevicius, 2019). Thorndike theorized that the cat learned to escape the cage by trial and error, where positive reinforcement was involved. Analysis of this experiment showed that the behavior that provided the desired effect became dominant and, therefore, occurred faster (Olencevicius, 2019).

Key Takeaways for Health Care Leaders

It can be asserted that feedback is requisite for providing both positive and negative reinforcement for behavior that is either desired or undesired. This handbook explores reinforcement theory in some detail (see Chapter 5 on

B. F. Skinner's reinforcement theory). Feedback creates the essential communication link between the behavior that is exhibited by the health care worker and the acknowledgement or recognition of that behavior by the health care manager, and provides either positive or negative reinforcement to the health care worker. Therefore, feedback is the communication message the health care manager provides the health care worker as it pertains to the worker's behavior, including effort and performance.

Feedback is something most health care workers seek from their supervisor, as well as from their coworkers, patients, families, and others in management. In addition, health care managers—just like other health care workers—also seek feedback from their supervisor, coworkers, and others. Above all, feedback provided by the supervisor to the health care worker may just be the most important feedback of all. Why? Because it is the supervisor who is typically responsible for the supervisory functions that impact the health care worker's employment status and working relationship, including staffing; assigning shifts, tasks, or duties; completing and administering performance evaluations; and providing periodic increases in compensation. In addition, the health care worker's supervisor typically has a significant impact on the employee's level of motivation and engagement, tenure, and even potential for promotion. As the old saying goes:

> Feedback is the breakfast of champions.

However, feedback is time sensitive. Feedback is most effective in the moment and loses its luster of effectiveness over time. Feedback is different than performance evaluation, where the latter is typically provided at the end of a set time period, such as a 90-day probationary period, or 12-month performance appraisal or evaluation period. Evaluation is typically communication provided by a health care manager to a subordinate regarding the subordinate's performance on a number of different performance or evaluation criteria or areas over the set time period.

A majority of health care workers want their supervisor—as well as coworkers and others—to provide them with feedback on a periodic, regular, or routine basis.

As a health care leader, make a habit of providing your subordinates with feedback on a periodic, regular, or routine basis regarding the work they are doing and its importance.

Be sure to include feedback relating to the health care worker's effort as well as performance.

Some employees want and need more feedback than others. As a health care manager, you need to understand which subordinates need and want more feedback versus those that don't, including the frequency of feedback, and provide subordinates feedback accordingly.

Some health care workers will be more sensitive to feedback they perceive as negative. It is the job of the health care manager to know their employees at a level where they can provide direct feedback in a way that is constructive. Moreover, health care managers need to choose their words carefully when providing feedback. The point is to provide appropriate feedback that is direct, specific, and to the point, and understandable, but professional, respectful, and constructive, and that doesn't offend or anger. Most health care workers can accept negative or constructive feedback when it is delivered in a professional and caring manner, represents the truth, and is still supportive and encouraging.

Ken Blanchard and Paul Hersey published situational leadership theory in their bestselling 1969 book, *Management of Organizational Behavior: Utilizing Human Resources*. The concept of situational leadership suggests that health care managers need to manage their employees differently depending on the employee's job readiness (knowledge, skill, ability, and experience doing the job or work) and psychological readiness (level of motivation to do the job). For example, a registered nurse (RN) who is a recent graduate with minimal experience will need more on-the-job training, coaching, and direction than an RN with 10 years of experience, in general and with all things being equal.

As a health care manager, choose the opportunity or medium for feedback that produces the impact and results you desire. For example, feedback can be in person, via email, text message, letter, handwritten note, or a second person. Feedback can also be provided in private to the respective health care worker, or in a public setting in front of others, such as at a staff meeting or other forum. As a rule, feedback should be provided in a medium or environment that is appropriate for the type of feedback, the sensitivity of the employee, and the relationship the health care manager has with the health care worker.

Health care managers should consider utilizing the Hawthorne effect when providing feedback intervention while employing management by walking around (or administrative rounds), observing, and interacting with health care workers in action. For example, when a health care leader acknowledges and extends their thanks and appreciation to health care workers, such as nurses, for providing direct patient care, the leader can highlight the good work nurses are doing and the difference they are making. This simple act of leadership can be very motivating to employees. Moreover, the health care leader can also explain how the nurses' work is positively impacting patients and patient care, the work of other employees, the department's pursuit of its objectives or goals, attainment of the mission and vision of the organization, and the overall improvement of the health status of the community at large. Moreover, it is important for health care managers to periodically provide health care workers feedback in context of their employee's dependability, reliability, creativity, problem-solving, initiative, teamwork, and other important work-related intangibles they are demonstrating. Overall, feedback can be one method used to help health care workers see and understand how the valuable work they do is in support of the organization's mission of patient care, as well as other important goals, helping them feel a stronger sense of worth, contribution, and connection to the organization as well as their overall motivation.

When used appropriately, feedback is also a method which can strengthen the supervisor–subordinate relationship. Moreover:

> Feedback can increase an employee's job satisfaction, employment relationship, and, consequently, their desire to stay with the organization (retention) and be motivated to provide the organization with the best they have to give.

Examples of Positive and Constructive In-Person Feedback

Examples of positive in-person, face-to-face, direct feedback given well by a health care leader include (a) recognizing and acknowledging the good work the employee is doing; (b) emphasizing one or two specific tasks, activities, or accomplishments of the employee; and (c) praising the employee for one or more intangibles they consistently demonstrate, such as dependability, reliability, hard work, working overtime when needed, and support of and collaboration with teammates. Examples of constructive in-person, face-to-face feedback given well includes providing feedback in private setting and (a) thanking the employee for the work they are doing, but identifying what specifically they could improve upon and why this is important; (b) providing the employee with thoughts and suggestions regarding how they could make the specific improvements; and (c) offering support and encouragement to the employee for making the improvements needed, and highlighting the difference the improvements will make for the employee, their colleagues, the patients and families, and the organization.

LEADERSHIP ACTION STEPS FOR FEEDBACK INTERVENTION

1. Feedback must be authentic, accurate, honest, and, as a general rule, based on firsthand observation or knowledge. While feedback can be given based upon secondhand information, the health care manager must be 100% sure the feedback is accurate.
2. A health care manager should ask subordinates (individually) about feedback and their expectations and preferences for same, including mediums, frequency, and so on.
3. As a general rule, a health care manager can provide positive feedback in both a private and public setting, but negative feedback should almost always be provided in a private setting. Generally, negative feedback tends to be more personal and private in nature and should therefore be treated accordingly.

4. As a general rule, if the health care manager isn't sure of what medium the feedback should be provided in, it is best to provide the feedback in person, face-to-face, in a private setting.
5. A health care manager should use the concept of situational leadership as a consideration in providing feedback. A health care manager must know and understand the job readiness and psychological readiness of each subordinate in order to be effective and appropriate with feedback, including mediums and frequency.

Assessing One's Leadership Style and Feedback Intervention

The following questions are designed to prompt reflection and self-assessment, and to promote better understanding and insight about how you—as a student, health care manager, or leader—can use or are using feedback intervention with your own leadership style. Use the following 5-point Likert scale for this assessment:

5 = Always 4 = Sometimes 3 = Neutral 2 = Seldom 1 = Rarely/Never

1. I routinely and consistently provide my subordinates with honest, accurate feedback that is encouraging and constructive, typically based upon my firsthand observations.

   5 4 3 2 1

2. I ask subordinates individually about feedback and their expectations and preferences regarding mediums and frequency, and do so periodically in the event their expectations or preferences have changed.

   5 4 3 2 1

3. I routinely provide positive feedback in private or public mediums or environments as appropriate, but as a rule always provide negative feedback in a private setting.

5 4 3 2 1

4. I routinely utilize the situational leadership concept in providing feedback to subordinates, considering each subordinate's job readiness and psychological readiness.

5 4 3 2 1

5. I routinely employ management by walking around and provide subordinates with feedback that helps them connect the valuable work they do with the organization's mission and other related goals and objectives.

5 4 3 2 1

____

____

____

____

References

Blanchard, K., & Hersey, P. (1969). *Management of organizational behavior: Utilizing human resources*. Prentice-Hall.

Cherry, K. (2023, September 28). Edward Thorndike's Contributions to Psychology. Verywell Mind. https://www.verywellmind.com/edward-thorndike-biography-1874-1949-2795525

Olencevicius, S. (2019). Feedback intervention research historical review: From single to multidimensional, *Journal of Contemporary Management Issues*, *24*, 55–69.

Reed, S. B. (2018). *Becoming a healthcare leader*. Cognella Academic Publishing.

Thorndike, E. L. (1911). Classics in the History of Psychology — Thorndike (1911) Chapter 5. Psychclassics.yorku.ca. https://psychclassics.yorku.ca/Thorndike/Animal/chap5

CHAPTER 4

Maslow's Hierarchy of Needs Theory

Have you ever worked through lunch on a busy workday because you weren't able to stop or take time to eat, and by midafternoon you were getting really hungry and becoming almost preoccupied with getting something to eat? One of our most basic needs for survival is food, and working hard requires nutrients from food for us to maintain our energy and overall health. Therefore, if we skip a meal and get hungry, we will probably become more motivated by getting something to eat rather than being concerned with self-actualizing or reaching our highest level of performance potential for that moment or time. This is the concept of Maslow's hierarchy of needs theory—we focus on and are motivated by our most basic needs that relate to survival, such as food, safety, security, and shelter when these needs are unsatisfied, but will focus on and be more motivated by higher-level needs, such as belonging, esteem, achievement, and self-actualization, once our more basic needs have been satisfied.

Background and Overview

Maslow's hierarchy of needs theory is one of the more commonly recognized motivational theories, and has been around for well over half a century. In 1943, American psychologist Abraham Maslow published a paper titled "*A Theory of Human Motivation*" in the journal *Psychological Review*, and then subsequently added to this body of work later. Maslow's framework is visually depicted in a pyramid, with the most basic needs (or deficiency needs) represented at the bottom of the pyramid and the higher-order needs (or growth needs) highlighted towards the top. According to Maslow's theory, a person must meet or somewhat substantially fulfill all the basic needs first before moving onto the pursuit of higher-order needs. Moreover, a person must have substantially fulfilled all the needs below in the pyramid before becoming motivated to pursue self-actualization, the highest-level need of all, that sits on top of the pyramid. However, Maslow suggested that a certain need would dominate a person's motivation at any given time, which recognizes that different levels of motivation could occur at any moment in time.

Maslow stated that "what you can become, you must become" (Maslow cited in Thompson, 2023).

> "One's only rival is one's own potentialities. One's only failure is failing to live up to one's own possibilities."
>
> (Maslow cited in Thompson, 2023).

It is interesting to note that the pyramid itself was not part of Maslow's original work, but came later as a way to graphically display the theory, providing greater ease of understanding by its visual representation.

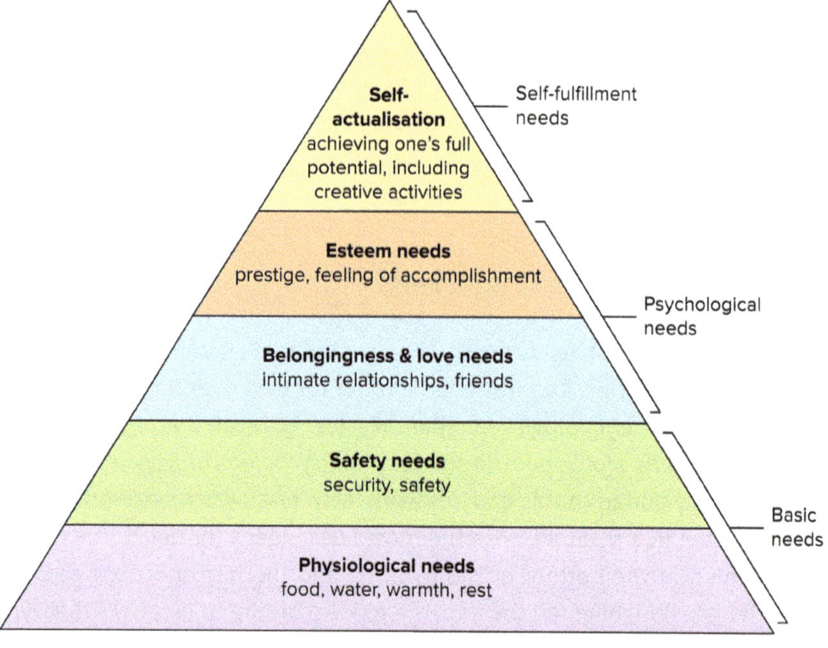

Figure 4.1 Maslow's Hierarchy of Needs

As depicted above at the bottom of Maslow's pyramid, physiological needs are the most basic of all needs and include food, water, air, shelter, sleep, clothing, and the like. Safety needs are next and include health, personal security, emotional security, and financial security. Belongingness and love needs are next and include family, friendship, trust, acceptance, affection, love, and intimacy. Esteem needs are next and include self-respect, self-confidence, respect from others, admiration from others, attention from others, and freedom and independence. And finally, at the top of the pyramid are self-fulfillment needs, which include creativity, curiosity, foresight, and self-actualization. Self-actualization is when a person reaches (or substantially reaches) their highest level of potential, and includes partner acquisition; parenting; utilizing talents, gifts, and abilities to their fullest; and pursuing and achieving meaningful goals and purpose in life. While over time there have been adaptations and refinements to Maslow's hierarchy of needs theory, this is the classical version.

There have been several criticisms of Maslow's theory, including that levels in the hierarchy actually overlap one another and aren't necessarily separate and distinct. Maslow's ideas were further described in his 1954 book, *Motivation and Personality*, and then later modified by Clayton Alderfer's ERG theory, which is covered in Chapter 15 in this handbook. In addition, David McClelland proposed a need theory that featured three dominant needs that underpin human behavior—the need for achievement, power, and affiliation. Nevertheless, Maslow's theory has application for health care managers at any level of leadership responsibility in a hospital or health care organization.

Health Care Leaders Should Focus on Helping Individual Employees Achieve Their Goals

Health care leaders should work to understand the performance potential of their employees as well as their goals, expectations, and aspirations, and work to promote and foster the attainment of those individual goals, expectations, and aspirations. Health care leaders should also pay attention to the intrinsic value the work an employee is doing and providing them. Moreover, health care leaders should look for opportunities to support, accentuate, or expand upon these intrinsic values or attributes of the work that are providing internal satisfaction and reward to the employee. In some cases, the employee may have greater potential to learn, grow, and develop their skills and abilities and expand their contributions to patients, coworkers, the department, or organization. In essence, health care leaders who help their employees achieve their goals are promoting employee motivation, satisfaction, and fulfillment; fostering employee retention; and helping to reduce employee burnout as they support their employees moving towards self-actualization—the highest-order need of all on Maslow's hierarchy.

Key Takeaways for Health Care Leaders

Health care managers should expect the needs of health care workers to differ from one worker to another. Moreover, health care managers should expect the needs of health care workers to change over time.

> Health care managers need to ask health care workers about their needs periodically and try to fully understand the importance and meaning of those needs for each respective subordinate, as well as for teams collectively.

Furthermore, a health care manager needs to understand their own needs, the relative importance of each one, and the most appropriate and effective way to satisfy each one.

LEADERSHIP ACTION STEPS FOR MASLOW'S HIERARCHY OF NEEDS THEORY

1. Health care managers should create an environment where basic, lower-order needs of health care workers are continually and consistently being met. This includes creating a working environment where health care workers feel safe and secure and are provided with appropriate resources, including personal protective equipment that protects them from infections and contagious diseases that can be transmitted from patients and others.

2. Health care managers need to create an environment where all health care workers feel free to speak their mind and offer their opinion and suggestions without fear of personal judgment, ridicule, condemnation, or reprisal.
3. Health care managers need to make sure subordinates' work schedules accurately reflect the appropriate days/shifts/times they are to work, and that worker compensation is accurate and reflects all hours worked as well as nonproductive hours that should be paid.
4. Health care managers should create an environment where health care workers have ready access to clean air, healthy food, clean drinking water, coffee, snacks, and appropriate areas where they can eat and take breaks from the demands of their work. Occasional surprise refreshments for health care workers go a long way to not only help meet physiological needs, but also needs for belonging, appreciation, and respect.
5. Health care managers should always be honest and trustworthy. Health care managers need to be good listeners and empower their employees by providing them with as much freedom and autonomy as possible, allowing them to use their creativity to help problem-solve and improve individual and organizational efficiency and performance.
6. Health care managers need to make sure every employee is involved and engaged in their work and understand how it impacts and contributes to the team as well as others in the organization, including patients.
7. Health care managers should recognize the good work their employees and teams are doing, and clearly highlight how that work contributes to quality patient care, patient experience and satisfaction, teamwork and organizational goals, mission, and vision. Moreover, health care managers must provide regular feedback, as well as periodically express how the employee contributes to and is a vital part of the health care team that is positively impacting lives and the community being served. Building a spirit of teamwork and collaboration is also important and can include company culture training and company-sponsored functions that bring employees and teams together.

8. Health care workers should get to know and understand each employee and their goals, potential, and performance capabilities and look for opportunities, tasks, and projects where the employee can work towards achieving important objectives and demonstrate their individual potential as well as their ability to significantly contribute to a team. Employee training, career coaching, mentoring, creative and challenging projects and assignments, and leadership inspiration to move beyond the employee's comfort zone can all help the employee to feel empowered and move their efforts and contributions closer to their highest potential.

(Mack, n.d.; McLeod, 2024)

Assessing One's Leadership Style and Maslow's Hierarchy of Needs Theory

The following questions are designed to prompt reflection and self-assessment, and to promote better understanding and insight about how you—as a student, health care manager, or leader—can use/ or are using Maslow's hierarchy of needs theory with your own leadership style. Use the following 5-point Likert scale for this assessment:

5 = Always 4 = Sometimes 3 = Neutral 2 = Seldom 1 = Rarely/Never

1. I routinely and consistently work to make sure my subordinates' basic needs of safety and security are being met in their working environment, and that they have all the necessary training, coaching, and resources to keep themselves, their coworkers, and their patients safe.

5 4 3 2 1

2. I routinely and consistently work to make sure my subordinates' basic needs for coffee, tea, cold drinking water, snacks and refreshments, and an appropriate break area are being met and to help foster camaraderie. Moreover, I work to make sure my subordinates can consistently get their needed breaks and lunch period away from the demands of work and recognize the importance for same.

5 4 3 2 1

3. I routinely and consistently keep my promises, don't make promises I can't keep, and respectfully tell the truth which my subordinates can always count on.

5 4 3 2 1

4. I routinely and consistently provide my subordinates and teams with as much freedom and autonomy in their work as possible, making sure they have clear direction, support, and understanding of my expectations for their effort and performance.

5 4 3 2 1

5. I routinely and consistently solicit suggestions and ideas from my subordinates and teams and utilize and implement as many of them as possible, providing positive feedback and recognition for their efforts and contributions and the impact those are making.

5 4 3 2 1

- List two or three of the most frequent ways you do this, and indicate how your subordinates typically react:
  - A.
  - B.
  - C.

6. I get to know and fully understand my subordinates and their values, goals, needs, desires, and aspirations regarding their work and the working environment; provide them with support, coaching, and mentoring as needed; and provide them with as many opportunities as possible to demonstrate their performance capabilities while recognizing same.

5 4 3 2 1

____
____
____
____

References

Mack, S. (n.d.). Maslow's theory and approach to leadership style. *Chron.* Retrieved July 9, 2024, from https://smallbusiness.chron.com/maslows-theory-approach-leadership-style-71607.html

Maslow's hierarchy of needs. (2024). In *Wikipedia.* Retrieved July 9, 2024, from https://en.wikipedia.org/wiki/Maslow%27s_hierarchy_of_needs

McLeod, S. (2024, January 24). Maslow's Hierarchy of Needs. SimplyPsychology. https://www.simplypsychology.org/maslow.html

Thompson, G. (2023). 30 inspiring Abraham Maslow quotes to power-up your perspective. Achology. https://achology.com/psychology/30-abraham-maslow-quotes/

Creditlines

Fig. 4.1: Copyright © by Androidmarsexpress (CC BY-SA 4.0) at https://commons.wikimedia.org/wiki/File:Maslow%27s_Hierarchy_of_Needs2.svg.

CHAPTER 5

Burrhus Frederic (B. F.) Skinner's Reinforcement Theory of Motivation

During both my undergraduate and graduate education, as well as my administrative residency training as a hospital administrator, I learned that being visible in the organization and management by walking around (MBWA)—also referred to as making administrative rounds throughout the facility—was important. Believing versus appreciating the importance of being visible and MBWA are two different things. It wasn't until I become a hospital chief executive officer that I realized the importance of administrative visibility and being present with employees, especially being visible and connecting with them in their work areas when making administrative rounds. It was when I was out in the hospital, interacting with physicians and health care workers and observing the work and caring they displayed, that I began to truly appreciate the role each health care worker played in pursuit of the hospital's mission of providing great care and healing to every patient and family. And I noticed that the more visible I was in the hospital making administrative rounds, the more positive feedback I was receiving. The positive feedback helped reinforce the importance of my being visible and accessible to employees throughout the hospital on a regular basis, and motivated me to continue the practice and make it a priority as part of my ongoing busy schedule. The positive reinforcement I was receiving that was motivating me to conduct administrative rounds with regularity is what Skinner's reinforcement theory of motivation would say is "*the presentation of a stimulus contingent on a behavior that results in an increased frequency of that behavior in the future*" (Zola, 2022). Simply stated:

Behavior is influenced by its consequences.

Background and Overview

Burrhus Frederic (B. F.) Skinner was an American psychologist, behaviorist, author, inventor, and social philosopher who is considered the father of behaviorism. Skinner was a professor of psychology at Harvard University from 1958 until 1974. Skinner's reinforcement theory of motivation is also referred to as operant conditioning, which suggests that learning behavior change is the result of reinforcement or punishment, or that behavior is determined by its consequences. Skinner's work was based on Thorndike's law of effect, which suggested that behavior that is followed by pleasant consequences is more likely to be repeated, and behavior following by unpleasant consequences is less likely to be repeated (McLeod, 2018). In other words, reinforcement helps strengthen a response and makes it more likely that the behavior will occur again in the future. Consequences help to eliminate or reduce the likelihood that a behavior will occur again in the future.

Skinner suggested there are four types of operant conditioning techniques:

1. **Positive reinforces: the addition of a reward**. Examples of a reward could be anything from positive feedback or recognition to being delegated more authority, given a promotion, or even provided with an award, bonus, or increase in compensation.
2. **Negative reinforces: the removal of a punishment**. Examples of removal of punishment could be anything from the supervisor no longer requiring closer supervision and monitoring of the subordinate and their work effort and performance, to ending a probationary period whereby the subordinate was required to complete certain tasks, exhibit certain behaviors, or exhibit a specific level of performance in a specified time period, and now has been placed back into good standing.
3. **Positive punishers: the addition of a punishment**. Examples of the addition of punishment could include closer supervision and monitoring of the subordinate and their work effort and performance by the supervisor, or starting a probationary period whereby the subordinate is required to complete certain tasks, exhibit certain behaviors, or exhibit a specific level of performance within a specified timeframe in order to be placed back in good standing in their employment or not receive any further disciplinary action.

4. **Negative punishers: the removal of a reward**. Examples of the removal of a reward could be anything from the subordinate no longer receiving positive feedback or recognition from the supervisor to no longer being delegated more authority, freedom, or control in their job; being demoted from a temporary position of greater authority; or no longer being awarded a bonus or increase in compensation.
("Skinner's reinforcement theory," n.d.)

Skinner suggested that leadership is a learned behavior that is influenced by a person's genetics. This idea of leadership involving both nature (the individual traits, characteristics, and personality an individual is born with) and nurture (the education, training, and experience an individual receives) is Skinner's answer to the age-old question, *Are leaders born or made*? Skinner believed effective leaders possess a combination of inherited traits and characteristics, as well as learned behaviors through education, training, and/or experience. Skinner also believed that leaders must display hard work and determination to be effective, as captured in one of his more famous quotes:

> "A failure is not always a mistake; it may simply be the best one can do under the circumstance. The real mistake is to stop trying."
>
> (Thompson, 2023)

Follow-Up Is One Important Way a Health Care Leader Can Provide Reinforcement

An example of how reinforcement theory can be used to provide consequences is by fostering accountability through leadership follow-up with an employee. Let's say a particular health care worker doesn't typically complete tasks or assignments on time without some ongoing encouragement, prodding, or motivation by leadership. Furthermore, let's say the health care worker has been delegated an important assignment that needs to be completed on time by their health care leader. Moreover, the health care leader knows they must follow up periodically with this worker to provide the encouragement, oversight, prodding, and motivation needed for them to complete the important assignment on time. Without this leadership follow-up, the worker wouldn't typically complete the assignment on time, believing there would be no positive or negative consequences for her if she didn't.

Key Takeaways for Health Care Leaders

As noted above, positive reinforcement can include many things, some of which we might consider small things and some we might consider more substantial, more important, more meaningful, or more valuable. Two things are important to include here: (a) whether the type of positive reinforcement is appropriate for the given behavior, and (b) how the positive reinforcement is carried out or delivered. Skinner stated:

> "The way positive reinforcement is carried out is more important than the amount."
>
> (Thompson, 2023)

Positive feedback and recognition always seem appropriate. However, equity theory suggests that employees compare things like their compensation, treatment, and other employment factors to that of their coworkers and ask this question: *Am I being treated fairly and equitably regarding such factors as my compensation, treatment, opportunities provided, recognition, and support as compared to my coworkers*? Therefore, equity theory suggests that health care workers will consider whether the type and frequency of positive feedback they receive from their supervisor is fair, equitable, and consistent with that received by their coworkers and colleagues for similar behaviors (World of Work Project, 2019). (Equity Theory is discussed in more detail in Chapter 9 in this handbook.) Additionally, as suggested by Skinner, a health care manager needs to not just be thoughtful and careful about the type and frequency of positive feedback they provide to subordinates, but *how* they provide or deliver the positive feedback. For example, providing positive feedback to a subordinate in a private, one-on-one situation or setting—such as in the health care manager's office—is different than delivering the same positive feedback in a staff meeting in front of the subordinate's coworkers and peers. In general, providing feedback and recognition to subordinates as well as coworkers and colleagues that is timely and appropriate is desirable and encouraged; however, it must also be done in a way that will be viewed positively and as appropriate by all (or at least not viewed negatively).

Positive punishers or the addition of a punishment should be viewed in the same fashion regarding the appropriateness of how it is provided and delivered, as well as whether it will be perceived as fair and just. One important note here:

> As a general rule of thumb, it is good to praise or acknowledge the work of others publicly, while negative or constructive feedback should be delivered in private.

Another important aspect of applying Skinner's reinforcement theory of motivation that should be considered has to do with past practices or precedent, as well as the organization's culture. Precedent relates to how reinforcement has been applied in the past by the health care manager, and whether the application of reinforcement is being appropriately and consistently applied. In addition, what is expected, desired, and observed throughout the department and organization relative to its culture of reinforcement must also be taken into consideration. While it may be appropriate for a given health care manager to apply reinforcement more enthusiastically, frequently, or aggressively than other managers typically do in the organization, they should stay within the written and unwritten as well as spoken and unspoken parameters dictated by company policy and organization culture.

It is also important for a health care manager to be authentic and follow through with any reinforcement efforts that they might have indicated or even hinted at with a subordinate. As mentioned in a number of different ways in this handbook, a health care manager's credibility and trustworthiness is so very critical to their overall effectiveness as a leader. A leader has to be believable at their word in order to maintain a high level of credibility with health care workers they supervise, as well as with coworkers and colleagues throughout the organization. Simply put, as a health care leader, make sure you have the authority and ability to do what you say before you say it. And if you say you will do something, then do it.

LEADERSHIP ACTION STEPS FOR B. F. SKINNER'S REINFORCEMENT THEORY OF MOTIVATION

Step 1: The health care manager uses management by objectives (MBO) to collaboratively set goals and objectives for actions and behaviors with a subordinate.

Step 2: The health care manager determines the appropriate ways to reinforce the desired actions and behaviors of the subordinate, as well as negatively reinforcing the undesired actions and behaviors, if appropriate.

Step 3: The health care manager chooses procedures or leadership methods/techniques for changing actions and behaviors of the subordinate, as appropriate.

Step 4: The health care manager implements the procedures or leadership methods/techniques for changing actions and behaviors while monitoring or even recording the results.

Assessing One's Leadership Style and Skinner's Reinforcement Theory of Motivation

The following questions are designed to prompt reflection and self-assessment, and to promote better understanding and insight about how you—as a student, health care manager, or leader—can use or are using Skinner's reinforcement theory of motivation with your own leadership style. Use the following 5-point Likert scale for this assessment:

5 = Always 4 = Sometimes 3 = Neutral 2 = Seldom 1 = Rarely/Never

1. I routinely collaborate with subordinates to establish goals and objectives for desired actions, behaviors, performance, and results for subordinates.

   5 4 3 2 1

2. I routinely and consistently acknowledge, recognize, and reward my subordinates for the work they do and the contributions they are making, consistent with precedent and organizational culture.

5 4 3 2 1

- List two or three of the most frequent ways you do this:
  A.
  B.
  C.

3. I appropriately take into account past practices and precedent, equity theory, organizational culture, and my level of authority before providing or delivering reinforcement of any kind to subordinates.

5 4 3 2 1

4. I don't mention or hint at reinforcement until I have made sure I have the authority to provide or deliver the reinforcement, and it is appropriate given the behavior.

5 4 3 2 1

5. I am authentic when delivering reinforcement, and follow through with any reinforcement that I have mentioned or hinted at to a subordinate.

5 4 3 2 1

____

____

____

____

References

McLeod, S. (2018). Operant conditioning: what it is, how it works, and examples. Simply Psychology. https://www.simplypsychology.org/operant-conditioning.html

Skinner's reinforcement theory in the classroom. (n.d.). Teaching Channel. Retrieved July 25, 2024, from https://www.teachingchannel.com/k12-hub/blog/reinforcement-theory-classroom/

Thompson, G. (2023, June 27). 30 Thought-Provoking B. F. Skinner Quotes to Elevate your Perspective. Achology. https://achology.com/psychology/burrhus-frederic-skinner-quotes/

World of Work Project. (2019). Adams' equity theory of motivation: A simple summary. https://worldofwork.io/2019/02/adams-equity-theory-of-motivation/

Zola, A. (2022, May). What Is Reinforcement theory? WhatIs.com. https://www.techtarget.com/whatis/definition/reinforcement-theory

CHAPTER 6

Frederick Herzberg's Two-Factor Theory of Motivation

Have you ever received an increase in compensation relating to a new job, an annual performance evaluation, an annual cost-of-living adjustment, or a job promotion? Did you feel a sense of accomplishment, achievement, or satisfaction with the increase in compensation you received? An increase in compensation usually provides the recipient a sense of accomplishment, achievement, or satisfaction, along with a sense of fairness or equity based upon the situation. However, according to Frederick Herzberg, in most cases, these types of feelings associated with an increase in compensation may only last for a short time, and may not be motivational to any significant degree or have any real lasting impact or effect.

Background and Overview

Herzberg's two-factor theory of motivation is also called Herzberg's motivator-hygiene theory. According to Herzberg, compensation isn't really a motivator per se, but potentially a dissatisfier or demotivator that Herzberg called a hygiene factor. Herzberg labeled compensation as a hygiene factor because he believed that compensation really isn't truly a motivator, but a factor that can demotivate an employee if the employee doesn't feel that his compensation is fair, reasonable, or equitable.

Frederick Irving Herzberg was an American psychologist who later became professor of management at the University of Utah. Herzberg became very influential in business management, particularly with his introduction of job enrichment as well as the two-factor theory of motivation, which was first published in a book titled *The Motivation to Work* in 1959. Herzberg's theory was based upon research he conducted with two hundred engineers and accountants in Pittsburg, Pennsylvania, and then replicated by 16 additional studies, making the original study one of the most replicated studies ever in the field of job attitudes.

Herzberg's aim was to dissect employee attitudes regarding their job, and what impact those attitudes had on the person and their motivation towards their work. Herzberg's research was based upon two fundamental questions he asked the workers: (a) what pleased the workers about their job, and (b) what displeased workers about their job. What Herzberg concluded from his research was individuals had two separate and distinct sets of needs that Herzberg identified as either lower-level needs—to avoid pain and deprivation—which he called hygiene factors, and higher-level needs to grow psychologically—job content needs, intrinsic to the job itself, which he also called motivators. Herzberg suggested these factors are mutually exclusive in that meeting an individual factor is not tied or connected to any other factor, be it a hygiene factor or motivational factor. Furthermore, these factors are not opposites per se because they involve different sets of needs. For example, Herzberg states that "*the opposite of job satisfaction is not job dissatisfaction but, rather, no job satisfaction while the opposite of job dissatisfaction is not job satisfaction, but no job satisfaction*" (Herzberg, as cited in Render, 2019).

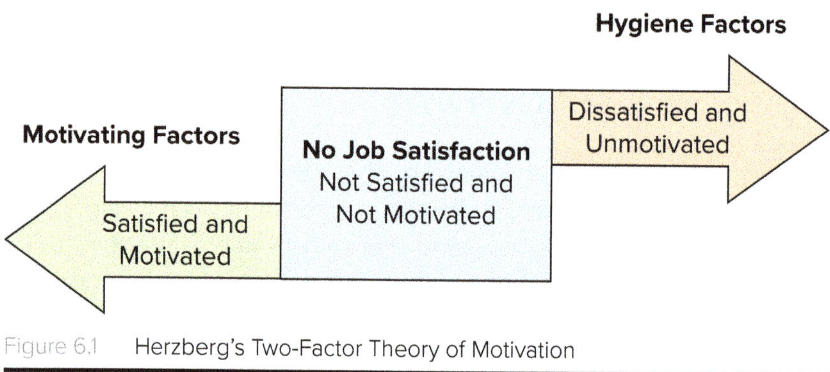

Figure 6.1 Herzberg's Two-Factor Theory of Motivation

Herzberg suggested that hygiene factors don't motivate employees or promote job satisfaction, but their absence can demotivate employees or prevent job satisfaction. The concept here is that good hygiene does not, in and of itself, produce good health; however, the lack of good hygiene can cause disease or infection. Herzberg suggested that motivational factors are the factors intrinsic to the job that can motivate employees, but their absence can also be demotivational. Here is a list of some of the factors in each of these two categories.

Hygiene Factors

- Compensation
- Benefits
- Comfortable work environment
- Reducing time spent at work
- Company policy and procedures
- Supervision
- Management scheduling
- Status
- Security
- Working relationships

Herzberg theorized that some hygiene factors require constant reinforcement to not be perceived or experienced as demotivators by employees.

Motivational Factors

- Achievement
- Recognition
- Satisfaction of the work itself
- Responsibility
- Opportunity
- Growth and development
- Self-scheduling
- Self-control of resources
- Self-accountability
- Empowerment

Herzberg's theory has some common themes with several other motivational theories discussed in this handbook, including the Hawthorne effect, Maslow's hierarchy of needs, and McGregor's Theory X and Theory Y.

Herzberg suggests to managers:

> "Forget praise. Forget punishment. Forget cash. You need to make their jobs more interesting."
>
> (Rau, 2023)

Much of the above information came from an article by Herzberg in the January 2003 issue of the Harvard Business Review, titled "*One More Time: How Do You Motivate Employees*?" In this article, Herzberg makes some interesting comments and observations that he refers to as "myths about motivation."

1. **Myth**: Reducing time spent on work will motivate employees.
   Reality: Motivated people seek more hours of work, not fewer.
2. **Myth**: Increasing wages motivates people.
   Reality: Yes—but only to seek the next wage increase.
3. **Myth**: Increasing fringe benefits motivates employees.
   Reality: Benefits are no longer viewed as rewards; they are viewed as rights.
4. **Myth**: Human relations training motivates employees.
   Reality: More human relations training has not resulted in more motivated employees.
5. **Myth**: Sensitivity training motivates employees to better understand and appreciate others.
   Reality: Only small, temporary gains have been achieved with sensitivity training.
6. **Myth**: Communication training motivates employees to better understand and appreciate others.
   Reality: No additional motivation has resulted from communication training.
7. **Myth**: Two-way communication activities between managers and employees improve communication and listening.
   Reality: Morale surveys and suggestion plans haven't improved motivation.
8. **Myth**: Job participation activities and providing employees with the bigger picture of their work motivates employees.
   Reality: Job participation activities haven't improved employee motivation.

9. **Myth**: Employee counseling programs improve employee motivation.
   Reality: Employee counseling has regained some momentum in the workplace recently but hasn't improved employee motivation.

Herzberg's central question throughout his (2003) article is, "*How do you install a generator in an employee?*"

Compensation Is a Short-Term Motivator

In health care today, there are growing manpower shortages in both clinical and nonclinical areas. Projections for future shortages in key health care disciplines can be described as foreboding. These manpower shortages have forced hospitals in competitive markets into a bidding war to recruit available personnel. Of course, this situation is principally driven by supply and demand, with the demand for health care manpower outweighing supply. Consequently, the argument can be made that compensation plays a more significant role today in the recruitment and retention of health care workers than in most previous time periods. However, it can also be argued—as asserted by Herzberg—that the intrinsic motivators of the job and work itself are more important and play a more significant role in employee satisfaction, motivation, and retention than compensation.

According to Herzberg, compensation is a hygiene factor and not a motivator. Therefore, when compensation for a given position is perceived as competitive as well as fair and equitable for the work being performed, then it won't be something viewed as a dissatisfier to the employee. However, in this situation it won't be a motivator either. Therefore, as a rule, compensation should generally be viewed as a short-term motivator at most. Therefore, a primary objective for hospitals and health service organizations when establishing compensation for various clinical and nonclinical positions should be for it to be perceived as competitive with the market, and fair and equitable internally for the skills, knowledge, and abilities required by the position.

Key Takeaways for Health Care Leaders

Herzberg's theory suggests that employee perception of a lack of sufficiency or adequacy in one or more hygiene factors will result in employees who are unhappy, demotivated, or dissatisfied with their job; who may exhibit lower effort and performance; or who might even consider quitting the organization altogether. On the contrary, when there is an employee perception of sufficiency or adequacy in motivational factors, then employees will be more motivated, more apt to be satisfied with their job, happier with the work and the company, and more likely to give greater effort and performance and to stay with the organization for a longer period. Motivating factors are job content factors—those things intrinsic to the job itself.

Herzberg suggests that an employee's work can be enriched to bring about greater employee motivation, including greater effort and performance. Job enrichment can provide opportunity for the employee's psychological growth, and greater satisfaction with the intrinsic values and rewards of the job. However, not all jobs can be enriched nor need to be enriched. When attempting to create job enrichment, Herzberg cautions managers not to add meaningless tasks to existing ones, to only rotate the same tasks or assignments, or remove difficult tasks of an assignment in order to free the worker to accomplish more of the less-challenging tasks or assignments: all of which Herzberg referred to as *horizontal loading* of a job.

LEADERSHIP ACTION STEPS FOR IMPROVING MOTIVATIONAL FACTORS

Herzberg (2003) suggests the following action steps to managers to create job enrichment, which is concomitant with improving motivational factors under Herzberg's theory.

1. Select jobs (to enrich) where existing attitudes are poor, hygiene is becoming costly, and motivation will make a difference in effort and performance.
2. Approach these jobs with the conviction that they can be changed. Move beyond the attitude of *but we've always done it this way*.
3. Brainstorm possible changes that may enrich these jobs.

4. Screen the list to remove suggestions that involve hygiene and not motivation.
5. Screen the list to remove suggestions that are too general and vague, typically accompanied by words such as *growth*, *achievement,* and *challenge*.
6. Screen the list to remove suggestions that are merely *horizontal loading* (see paragraph above).
7. Avoid having employees whose jobs will be enriched involved in making suggestions. It will be the content of the work that will produce motivation, not involvement in setting up the changes.
8. In the initial attempt, set up a controlled experiment. Chose two equivalent groups, with one having the motivators systematically introduced over a period of time, and the other group with no changes. Conduct pre- and post-installation tests of performance and attitudes and evaluate/assess impact.
9. Be prepared for a drop in performance in the experimental group, as changes to a new job may lead to a temporary reduction in efficiency.
10. Expect frontline supervisors to experience some anxiety and even hostility over the changes.

Assessing One's Leadership Style and Herzberg's Two-Factor Theory of Motivation

The following questions are designed to prompt reflection and self-assessment, and to promote better understanding and insight about how you—as a student, health care manager, or leader—can use or are using Herzberg's two-factor theory of motivation with your own leadership style. Use the following 5-point Likert scale for this assessment:

5 = Always 4 = Sometimes 3 = Neutral 2 = Seldom 1 = Rarely/Never

1. I routinely and consistently check in with my subordinates about their level of satisfaction regarding hygiene factors, and make changes or improvements as needed.

   5 4 3 2 1

2. I routinely and consistently recognize my subordinates for the work they do and the contributions they are making.

5 4 3 2 1

3. I routinely and consistently provide my subordinates with opportunities to contribute, achieve, learn, and develop, and provide them with opportunities for growth through new experiences and challenges.

5 4 3 2 1

- List two or three of the most frequent ways you do this:
  A.
  B.
  C.

4. I routinely and consistently provide my subordinates with as much autonomy as possible, empowering them with as much control over resources and decision-making as possible.

5 4 3 2 1

5. I routinely and consistently look for opportunities to enrich employee jobs by providing them with new and additional responsibilities and challenges that will engender self-control, self-accountability, and professional growth and development, which allows me more time to focus on higher-level employee development and leadership activities.

5 4 3 2 1

References

Herzberg, F. (2003, January). One more time: How do you motivate employees? *Harvard Business Review*. https://hbr.org/2003/01/one-more-time-how-do-you-motivate-employees

Rau, J. (2023). It's Not Enough To Pay Your Employees More. Forbes. https://www.forbes.com/sites/johnrau/2023/01/11/in-todays-economy-getting-employee-compensation-right-is-necessary-but-insufficient/

Render, J. (2019, February 25). Herzberg's two-factor theory of motivation. Agile-Mercurial. https://agile-mercurial.com/2019/02/25/herzbergs-two-factor-theory-of-motivation/

Creditlines

Fig. 6.1: Source: https://agile-mercurial.com/2019/02/25/herzbergs-two-factor-theory-of-motivation/.

CHAPTER 7

The Hawthorne Effect

To this day, when I know that someone is paying attention or watching me carefully with intent to follow my effort or performance, I am always more motivated to give my best. While the importance of the activity I am doing probably makes some difference, the attention being paid by someone seems to make an impact on my level of motivation. Doesn't it for you? Maybe this reaction has something to do with a sense of pride and wanting to always show others my best side. Maybe this reaction has more to do with not wanting to look bad in someone else's eyes. And sometimes this reaction has to do with setting an example or modeling the way.

Background and Overview

The Hawthorne effect is a type of human behavior reactivity in which individuals modify one or more aspects of their behavior in response to their awareness of being observed. Furthermore, this change in behavior typically relates to an increase in the performance of individuals who are noticed, watched, and paid attention to by supervisors (Perera, 2023).

The phrase "the Hawthorne effect" was first coined in 1958 by Henry A. Landsberger when analyzing earlier experiments from 1924 to 1932 at the Hawthorne Works plant owned and operated by Western Electric in Cicero, Illinois, near Chicago.

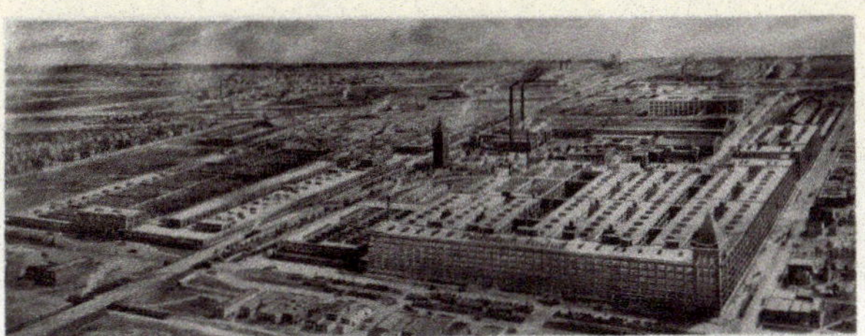

Figure 7.1 Hawthorne Works Plant

The Hawthorne Works plant was a large factory complex that was named after the original name of the town, Hawthorne. The plant opened in 1905 and operated until 1983. At its height in 1929, the Hawthorne Works plant had over 40,000 workers. The plant included offices, factories, a hospital, fire brigade, laundry facilities, and a greenhouse. Primarily the plant manufactured telephones, cable, telephone switching systems, and telephone equipment for AT&T. A set of studies or experiments was conducted at the Hawthorne Works plant in the 1920s by a team of two sociologists by the names of Roethlisberger and Whilehead, a psychologist by the name of Elton Mayo, and a company representative by the name William Dickson. There were four separate experiments conducted: (a) illumination experiments (1924 to 1927), (b) relay assembly test room experiments (1927 to 1932), (c) interviewing workers experiments (1928 to 1930), and (d) bank wiring room experiments (1931 to 1932). These experiments all pointed to one primary conclusion: The Hawthorne effect is a type of human behavior reactivity in which individuals modify one or more aspects of their behavior in response to their awareness of being observed. Furthermore, this change in behavior typically relates to an increase in the performance of individuals who are noticed, watched, and paid attention to by supervisors ("Hawthorne effect," n.d.).

> As the Hawthorne effect pertains to health care leadership, hospital and health service employees—both clinical and nonclinical alike—will generally be more motivated to improve their effort and performance when being noticed, acknowledged, recognized, observed in action, and/or paid attention to by their direct supervisor and/or other managers and leaders in the organization's hierarchy or chain of command.

Apply the Hawthorne Effect Through Management by Walking Around

One of the central themes of MBWA is for the health care leader to get out of their office, walk about in various areas and departments of the hospital or health service organization, be visible and pay attention to, observe, recognize, and interact with/engage with employees. While MBWA is not the only way, it can be one of the most effective ways for a health care leader to apply the Hawthorne effect. There is an old adage in leadership that says, *People don't care about what you know until they know you care*. Management by walking around is an effective way for health care leaders to demonstrate they care about their workers by visibly being out in the organization, observing and interacting with workers—in the workers' own work area or department—and displaying their attention and interest in the workers and the work they are doing. The time and attention health care leaders pay to health care workers in a direct, personal way such as this cannot be measured in terms of the positive impact it can have on employees and their overall satisfaction, employment relationship, and motivation.

Key Takeaways for Health Care Leaders

There has been some historical debate about how the studies at the Hawthorne Works plant were conducted, or even the results thereof. And while the experiments conducted at the Hawthorne Works plant in the 1920s and 1930s may be in the distant past, the Hawthorne effect itself has real, practical application for health care leaders looking to motivate health care employees to give of their effort and perform at a high level. Logic, common sense, and human nature all support the key point as noted above: As the Hawthorne effect pertains to health care leadership, hospital and health service employees—both clinical and nonclinical alike—will generally be more motivated to improve their effort and performance when being noticed, acknowledged, recognized, observed in action, and paid attention to by their direct supervisor or other leaders in the organization's hierarchy or chain of command.

LEADERSHIP ACTION STEPS FOR THE HAWTHORNE EFFECT

A majority of health care workers want a positive working relationship with their immediate supervisor. As a health care leader, get to know your employees, including their goals, motivators, demotivators, pet peeves, and their personality traits and characteristics, as well as their strengths, weaknesses, and potential for growth related to work. Health care leaders should pay attention to their workers.

A majority of health care workers want a relationship with a middle manager or senior leader, or to have at least one middle manager or senior leader to know what department or service they work in, and to call them by name when encountered. As a middle manager or senior leader, get to know employees by name and the department in which they work. As a frontline health care supervisor, work with your direct supervisor or other middle manager or senior leader, as appropriate, to be visible occasionally in your department and to learn the names of your employees and the work they do.

A majority of health care workers want the work they do to be acknowledged and recognized in some meaningful way by their immediate supervisor and even one or more other health care managers or senior leaders in the organization.

As a health care manager, always acknowledge your employees when seeing them in passing, as well as acknowledge their effort, performance, and contributions. Thank them periodically for all they do. Recognize employees during departmental staff meetings for their efforts and contributions.

A majority of health care workers want their immediate supervisor and even others on the management team to know and support them, and to understand and support their needs, goals, and aspirations. As a health care manager, go beyond just knowing and supporting your subordinates by taking the time and making the effort to clearly understand their goals and aspirations as a health care worker and to help them and support them in achieving their goals and aspirations. As a frontline health care manager, share some of the important goals and aspirations of your subordinates with your direct supervisor, another appropriate middle manager, or even with a senior leader, as appropriate. Just be sure to share job-related and work-related goals, as appropriate, with a supervisor or other manager that you might report to, as well as determine how your supervisor or other manager can help support your employees' efforts to achieve their goals.

A majority of health care workers appreciate it when their immediate supervisor checks in with them during the course of the workday/night, observes them doing their work, and offers help or support if needed. As a health care manager, this action is important because it shows you care and are concerned for your employees and the important work they are doing. Moreover, if you are in a position to jump in and help if needed, that also adds another element of support that can go a long way with your employees.

A majority of health care workers enjoy and appreciate it when someone from the management team or senior leadership makes rounds in their department and checks in with them about how they are doing, how things are going, observes them doing their work, and acknowledges and recognizes the good work they are doing. Health care leaders at all levels should periodically be making administrative rounds. As a general rule, frontline supervisors should typically make administrative rounds a regularly occurring activity in the daily work schedule. In contrast, senior leaders should be making administrative rounds weekly, biweekly, or at least monthly, depending on the size of the health care organization and the senior leader's position and responsibilities.

Many health care workers appreciate periodically receiving a handwritten note or card acknowledging and recognizing the efforts they make and the good work they are doing. To this point, there is really no substitute for a handwritten note versus an email. Will an email suffice? Yes, but an email is typically viewed as less personal in many regards than a handwritten note, which can have more of an impact on the receiver. I remember receiving a handwritten note from a previous supervisor thanking me for my hard work and efforts and recognizing the difference I was making. The handwritten note made me feel appreciated, supported, and inspired. I was a hospital chief operating officer of a 345-bed private, not-for-profit hospital at the time, and my supervisor was the chief executive officer.

Assessing One's Leadership Style and the Hawthorne Effect

The following questions are designed to prompt reflection and self-assessment, and to promote better understanding and insight about how you—as a student, health care manager, or leader—can use or are using the Hawthorne effect with your own leadership style. Use the following 5-point Likert scale for this assessment:

5 = Always 4 = Sometimes 3 = Neutral 2 = Seldom 1 = Rarely/Never

1. I routinely and consistently check in with my subordinates and observe them doing their work.

   5 4 3 2 1

2. I routinely and consistently acknowledge and recognize my subordinates for the work they do and the contributions they are making, including through giving handwritten notes or cards of praise and encouragement.

   5 4 3 2 1

- List two or three of the most frequent ways you do this:
  A.
  B.
  C.

3. I periodically help and assist with tasks of my employees to model the way and provide my support and encouragement to subordinates.

   5 4 3 2 1

4. I make it known outside my department or service area the good work my subordinates are doing and how they are contributing to patient care delivery, quality outcomes, patient experience, and the organization's mission.

    5   4   3   2   1

5. I make administrative rounds (management by walking around or MBWA) frequently and consistently to be visible and accessible, to demonstrate my interest and concern for my subordinates, and to engage with them appropriately.

    5   4   3   2   1

____

____

____

____

References

Hawthorne effect. (n.d.). In *Wikipedia.* Retrieved July 9, 2024, from https://en.wikipedia.org/wiki/Hawthorne_effect

Perera, A. (2023, February 8). Hawthorne effect: Definition, how it works, and how to avoid it. *Simply Psychology.* https://www.simplypsychology.org/hawthorne-effect.html

Reed, S. B. (2018). *Becoming a healthcare leader.* Cognella Academic Publishing.

Creditlines

Fig. 7.1: Western Electric Company, https://commons.wikimedia.org/wiki/File:Hawthorne,_Illinois_Works_of_the_Western_Electric_Company,_1925.jpg, 1925.

CHAPTER 8

Douglas Murray McGregor's Theory X and Theory Y

Have you ever described, or had someone else describe, a manager's leadership style in one word? Think about it: Can a one-word description of a manager's leadership style really convey a lot of meaning? In the case of the following one-word description, it is typically informative and descriptive of a manager's leadership style that is unfortunately all too common, and generally has a very negative connotation. The word is *micromanager*. This word has been used to describe numerous leaders at various levels of management who are overly controlling, highly directive, and generally don't trust workers to take responsibility and get the job done right without a lot of direct supervision. These are leaders who are supervising employees so closely they have created a work environment where employee dissatisfaction is high; creativity, innovation, and motivation are low; and there is probably significant turnover as employees are looking for a better working environment altogether. So what type of leadership philosophy or style does a micromanager typically espouse?

A micromanager is typically a manager who believes in Theory X as described by Douglas McGregor. Theory X and Theory Y are two contrasting theories developed and promulgated by Douglas McGregor about what a manager might assume or believe about employees as it relates to their work ethic and psychological motivation to work. And a manager's assumptions or beliefs about the work ethic and psychological motivation of employees significantly impacts their leadership style.

Background and Overview

Douglas McGregor was an American social psychologist, professor at MIT Sloan School of Management, and president of Antioch College from 1948 to 1954. McGregor first promulgated his two theories—Theory X and Theory Y—in his book *The Human Side of Enterprise*, published in 1960. McGregor's book was voted the fourth most influential management book of the 20th century in a poll of the Fellows of the Academy of Management ("Douglas McGregor," 2024). In his book, McGregor starts by asking the following simple yet thought-provoking question:

> "What are your assumptions (implicit as well as explicit) about the most effective way to manage people?"
>
> (McGregor, 2006)

McGregor suggested that a manager's individual assumptions about human nature and behavior determined how that individual would manage their employees. Managers who are more inclined to assume or believe their employees dislike their work, have little motivation, and don't want to take or shouldn't take responsibility, fall into the Theory X category. These are managers who take a more pessimistic view of employees and therefore tend to be more controlling, provide more direction, and are more inclined to closely supervise employees while typically not providing much autonomy or freedom, and tightly controlling decision-making. As previously stated, these types of managers are commonly referred to as *micromanagers*.

Managers who are more inclined to assume or believe their employees can be trusted, are motivated to do a good job, are self-directed, and can take on greater amounts of responsibility, fall into the Theory Y category. These are managers who take a more optimistic view of employees and therefore are much more participative in their management style. These managers provide employees with more autonomy and freedom; allow employees to seek and accept responsibility through delegation; and support employees and work collaboratively with them to solve problems and improve performance. Managers who espouse Theory Y to a great extent are commonly referred to as *hands-off* managers.

Health care managers who effectively espouse Theory Y in their leadership style tend to be empowering to their workers, as they typically delegate authority and decision-making to the lowest level possible, and allocate and equip employees with the knowledge, skills, and resources necessary to make and execute decisions effectively. Health care managers who effectively espouse Theory Y in their leadership style believe in employee empowerment (Reed, 2018).

> "Empowerment is creating feelings of intrinsic motivation in which employees perceive their work to have impact and meaning, and perceive themselves to be competent and capable of self-determination"
>
> *(Reed, 2018, p. 123).*

See Chapter 16, Julian Rappaport's Empowerment Theory of Motivation, for more information on this topic.

Health Care Leaders Need to Be Aware of Their Predilection for Theory X or Theory Y

Early career health care leaders—those with limited leadership experience—need to especially be intentional about being aware of their predilection for either Theory X or Theory Y, and how this philosophy or belief is showing up in their leadership style. Why? Without a health care leader's awareness and clear insight into their own natural inclination toward either Theory X or Theory Y, the leader may be following their natural predilection or inclination at times when they shouldn't. This is particularly true with early career and inexperienced leaders, because they don't have as much experience to fall back on, to remind them or make apparent to them situations or occasions where they should flex or adjust their leadership style away from what might come naturally—that is, from Theory X to Theory Y, or vice versa.

For example, an early career or inexperienced health care leader who has a natural proclivity towards Theory X may not provide the experienced, high-performing employee with as much autonomy as appropriate because the health care leader is relying on her natural proclivity to not trust the employee to the extent they should, or to not believe the employee will be as responsible as they would otherwise, or to not provide as much freedom or autonomy in general because of their Theory X philosophy or belief. Alternatively, an early career or inexperienced health care leader who has a natural proclivity towards Theory Y may provide a new, inexperienced, and marginally motivated employee with too much autonomy because the health care leader is relying on her natural proclivity to trust the employee to know everything they are doing. Moreover, the early career or inexperienced health care leader may also believe this employee will be totally responsible and can be provided with a significant amount of freedom or autonomy to do their work given the health care leader's Theory Y philosophy or belief—which isn't appropriate in this case either.

Key Takeaways for Health Care Leaders

Most managers probably have a predisposition for either Theory X or Theory Y, and both approaches can be motivational in their own right. However, situation leadership theory suggests that health care managers should use a mix of Theory X and Theory Y approaches, depending on the job readiness and psychological readiness of the respective health care worker (Center for Leadership Studies, n.d.) For example, a newly hired registered nurse who has just completed her education and training will likely need a management style that espouses Theory X—at least in the beginning period of her tenure. Inexperienced health care workers, by definition, will most likely need more supervision, direction, guidance, support, and coaching than experienced workers. Alternatively, experienced health care workers who are energetic; eager to do a good job; want to learn, grow, and contribute; and who are generally motivated to give good effort and perform well will need less supervision, direction, guidance, support, and coaching as a general rule. However, there are other factors that may impact or influence a health care manager's espousal and incorporation of Theory X and/or Theory Y into their leadership style that should be considered for a given situation, circumstance, or even individual health care worker.

A health care manager should be cognizant of each subordinate's respective attitudes about their work, their job, their career, and the organization, and realize these attitudes can change at any time due to a multitude of different factors, variables, and reasons.

Health care managers need to be aware regarding their own attitudes and beliefs about health care workers and their attitudes about work, including giving their effort, working hard, accepting responsibility, and being reliable and trustworthy.

Health care managers need to continually assess their own assumptions and beliefs about health care workers' human nature towards work, and how their attitudes towards work ethic manifest in their leadership philosophy and style.

Societal and cultural norms today suggest that Theory Y, overall and in general, is a more motivational approach towards managing health care workers. However, an organization's own culture towards managing employees, and autocratic versus decentralized decision-making (typically driven from senior leadership), will also be highly influential in which approach—Theory X or Theory Y, and to what degree and in what mix with employees—a manager might want or need to align their leadership style to in their current position (Mind Tools, n.d.).

LEADERSHIP ACTION STEPS FOR THEORY X AND THEORY Y

1. Health care managers should take time to periodically reflect, assess, and evaluate their own assumptions, attitudes, and inherent beliefs about health care workers' human nature and natural behaviors towards work and responsibility. Moreover, health care managers should assess and evaluate how these assumptions, attitudes, and inherent beliefs manifest in their respective leadership philosophy and style.
2. Health care managers should communicate openly and regularly with subordinates, inquiring about their perceptions regarding the work environment and the manager's leadership style. Health care managers need to shape and mold their leadership style appropriately based upon employee perceptions and feedback; however, they need to do so in context and compatibility with their overall leadership philosophy and the culture of the organization.

3. Health care managers should listen to subordinates' communication and observe their behaviors ongoing to assess their motivation to work, including their attitudes and behaviors towards taking responsibility, their coworkers, and the organization.
4. Health care managers should recognize that the majority of health care workers are working in health care to make a positive impact on the lives of others; therefore, as a general rule, health care workers generally seek responsibility and autonomy, and are self-directed and committed. As a result, health care managers should seek to empower health care workers to the greatest extent appropriate, which will create a more motivational work environment. However, situational leadership suggests there is always an appropriate time and place for using a Theory X approach.
5. Health care managers should recognize that today's societal and cultural norms favor a leadership style that is more Theory Y based. In general, most employees desire freedom, autonomy, self-direction, and empowerment from leadership. A health care manager who can incorporate and optimize these Theory Y leadership qualities effectively within the organizational culture of the company can provide a more motivational work environment that will foster employee effort and performance.

Assessing One's Leadership Style and Theory X and Theory Y

The following questions are designed to prompt reflection and self-assessment, and to promote better understanding and insight about how you—as a student, health care manager, or leader—can use or are using Theory X and Theory Y with your own leadership style. Use the following 5-point Likert scale for this assessment:

5 = Always 4 = Sometimes 3 = Neutral 2 = Seldom 1 = Rarely/Never

1. I periodically reflect, assess, and evaluate my own assumptions, attitudes, and inherent beliefs about health care workers' human nature and behaviors toward work and responsibility. Moreover, I assess and evaluate how these assumptions, attitudes, and inherent beliefs manifest in my own leadership philosophy and style.

   5 4 3 2 1

2. I routinely and consistently communicate openly and regularly with subordinates, inquiring about their perceptions regarding the working environment and my leadership style. I shape and mold my leadership style appropriately based upon employee perceptions and feedback, in context and compatibility with my overall leadership philosophy and the culture of my organization.

   5 4 3 2 1

3. I routinely and consistently listen to subordinates' communication and observe their behaviors ongoing to assess their psychological readiness and motivation to work, including their attitudes and behaviors towards work, taking responsibility, autonomy, and supervision.

   5 4 3 2 1

4. I empower my subordinates to the greatest extent appropriate to create a more motivational work environment. However, I follow situational leadership theory and use a Theory X approach as appropriate when and where indicated and needed.

   5 4 3 2 1

- List two or three of the most frequent ways you do this:
  - A.
  - B.
  - C.

5. I routinely and consistently assess and evaluate my organization's culture regarding providing worker autonomy and freedom; allowing workers to seek and accept responsibility through delegation and decentralized decision-making; and supporting workers and working collaboratively with them to solve problems and improve performance.

5 4 3 2 1

____

____

____

____

References

Center for Leadership Studies. (n.d.). Situational leadership. Retrieved July 9, 2024, from https://situational.com/situational-leadership/

"Douglas McGregor." (n.d.). In *Wikipedia*. Retrieved July 9, 2024, from https://en.wikipedia.org/wiki/Douglas_McGregor

McGregor, D. (2006) The Human Side of Enterprise, Annotated Edition. First edition ed., McGraw Hill.

Mind Tools. (n.d.). Theory X and Theory Y. Retrieved July 9, 2024, from https://www.mindtools.com/adi3nc1/theory-x-and-theory-y

Reed, S. B. (2018). *Becoming a healthcare leader.* Cognella Academic Publishing.

CHAPTER 9

John Stacey Adams's Equity Theory of Motivation

Am I compensated fairly as it relates to the work I do, and my efforts, contributions, and overall performance? Am I compensated fairly in comparison with my colleagues and coworkers? These are a few questions virtually every health care worker has on an ongoing basis. Furthermore, every health care worker will answer this question for themselves. Exactly how the employee answers these questions will impact their level of motivation—overall and at any given moment. It can be argued that as the health care labor market tightens in terms of health care manpower shortages relative to demand, this question of being compensated fairly in comparison with others may take on more significance than ever before. As hospitals and health care organizations find recruitment and retention more competitive than ever, organizations are increasingly competing on compensation with the growing imbalance in the supply and demand of health care manpower.

Background and Overview

John Stacey Adams was a workplace and behavioral psychologist. Adams developed the equity theory of motivation in 1963 to provide a theoretical explanation for the psychological basis of inequity perceived by employees working for private employers and government. Equity theory suggests there are two factors at play for employee motivation: (a) a perception that management or the organization is rewarding the employee fairly for the work they are doing and the contributions they are making, and (b) the perception that the employee's reward for the work and contributions they are making is also fair in terms of comparisons to other employees, the work they are doing, and rewards they are receiving. At its core, Adams's equity theory says that individuals want a fair relationship between inputs and outputs. Adams suggests that without this perception of fairness the employee will not be motivated and may even feel distressed and try to change things in some way to create a sense of balance or fairness (Davlembayeva & Alamanos, 2023).

The central theme or point of equity theory is fairness, and fairness is based upon a perception made by the employee about the work being done (an individual's inputs or contributions) and the compensation and other rewards (benefits, rewards, recognition, and compensation) being received—by themselves and in comparison to others. Inputs or contributions can take many different forms, such as time or hours worked, quality or effort put into the work, the type of work and its importance, contributions the work is making to the organization's operations, mission or goals, teamwork, problem-solving, loyalty, enthusiasm, support of others, and even ability to complete tasks autonomously. Outputs, benefits, recognition, and rewards include things such as compensation, bonuses, flexibility, trust, benefits, job security, job opportunities, stimulating work, education and training opportunities, promotion, recognition, appreciation, and praise or thanks. For a health care worker to feel things are fair and equitable, they need to feel the benefits they receive per unit of contribution are similar to the benefits that their peers, coworkers, and colleagues receive for a comparable unit of contribution. When the perception of fairness exists, the employee may be motivated; however, when there is a perception of unfairness, the health care worker may stop being motivated. The greater the degree of unfairness perceived, the greater the level of distress the health care worker may feel. This distress can manifest in feelings of unfairness, not being appreciated, or even humiliation, anger, or injustice. Moreover, the health care worker most likely will attempt to return the situation to a state of fairness either by adjusting contributions he is making or adjusting the perception about how much he is contributing or its value.

There is the possibility that some health care workers may feel overcompensated, or that the outputs or rewards are greater than the work they are doing or the contributions they are making. Consequently, these health care workers may (a) look to increase their effort, performance, or contributions, or (b) adjust their perceptions of the relative value of the effort, performance, or contributions they are making, either consciously or subconsciously, through a process known as cognitive distortion. Moreover, the health care worker may use cognitive distortion by either inflating their perception of what they are contributing, or deflating their perception of what others are contributing (World of Work, 2019).

TEST 1:
The Equity of Reward and Input

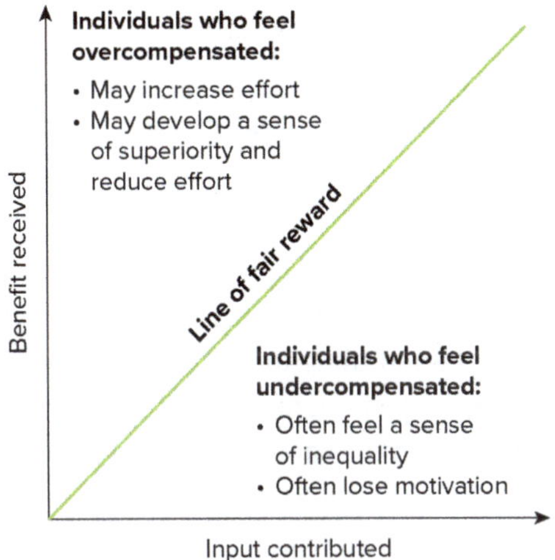

Figure 9.1a

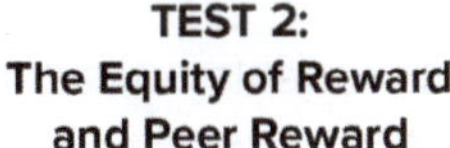

TEST 2:
The Equity of Reward and Peer Reward

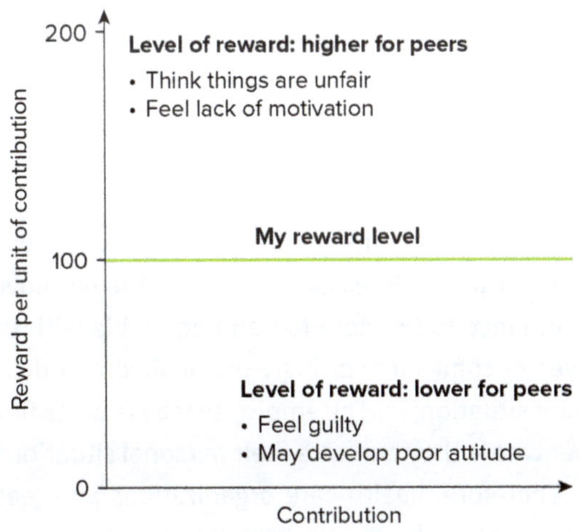

Figure 9.1b Adams's Equity Theory

Adams's equity theory is also applicable to teams or groups of health care workers. Since much of the work done in hospitals is through teams or departments, this is important for health care managers to consider when managing or leading teams or departments.

Adams's Equity Theory and Compensation Versus Effort and Performance

Isn't paying hourly health care workers the same hourly rate who work in the same job classification and have the same tenure or length of service with the organization the preferred thing to do? Adams's equity theory suggests the answer to this question just might be *maybe not*. Paying employees the same hourly rate who work in the same job classification and have the same tenure or length of service with the organization is a very common practice in health care, and probably the simplest and most efficient method of compensation for hourly workers. However, as suggested by equity theory, this common practice may also motivate those same employees to give similar effort and perform at a similar level to that of their coworkers and colleagues *regardless of whether some of those employees have much more to give and contribute.*

There are numerous variables or factors that can motivate employees capable of giving more of their effort and performing at a higher level, otherwise referred to as their discretionary effort. However, an employee's perception of their compensation relative to their coworkers' compensation, and their perceived effort and performance compared to that of their coworkers, will be viewed as either comparable, and therefore fair and equitable, or not. When an employee's perception of their compensation relative to their effort and performance as compared to that of their coworkers is viewed as not fair or equitable, several possibilities can result: (a) The employee lowers their effort and performance to be more fair and equitable with their coworkers; (b) The employee becomes increasingly dissatisfied and disenchanted with their employment situation; (c) The employee may leave to find another position or employer where they perceive their personal situation to be more fair and equitable. Therefore, health care organizations and leaders who have elected to pay hourly health care workers the same hourly rate who work in the same job classification and have the same tenure or length of service with the organization, regardless of their effort, performance, and contributions to the organization, may be overlooking how this is perceived by those hourly employees affected, particularly those who have more to give and contribute than they believe they are being paid for.

Key Takeaways for Health Care Leaders

Health care workers, like most people in general, value fair and equitable treatment by government, by society, by their supervisor at work, by coworkers and colleagues, and by family, friends, and others in most every aspect of their life. In particular, health care workers want fair and equitable treatment from their immediate supervisor as well as from the management team at large and the organization in general.

Health care workers will look to many things regarding their treatment and make a judgment as to whether that treatment is fair and equitable. Some of the more obvious and apparent things health care workers will look to regarding fairness and equitability are compensation, benefits, application of policies and procedures, performance appraisals, opportunities for promotion, and work assignments. Other considerations can include authorization for days off, feedback from their immediate supervisor, recognition, awards, or even how the supervisor reacts to health care worker suggestions, input, or feedback. Still other considerations can include job-related resources provided, support provided, advice or coaching provided, and even attention given, or direct communication or observation provided. Again, the health care worker will assess all these things—and more—based upon their own determination of fairness and equitability. Moreover, this assessment of fairness and equitability will be made—in part or in total—in comparison to treatment of coworkers and colleagues for the same or similar considerations (Mata et al., 2021).

There can also be many other variables at play in this equation. For example, variables at play can include the health care manager's leadership style in the past, and the health care worker's assessment of their treatment historically by the health care manager and possibly others on the management team. Other variables can include the treatment a health care worker received in a previous service or department, or by a previous coworker—all which can be factors at play in the worker's perception of fairness regarding their treatment and overall employment relationship.

A health care manager needs to really know and understand the overall psychological characteristics and makeup of his subordinates regarding things such as job and psychological readiness; need or desire for the manager's attention, support, advice, coaching, encouragement, praise, recognition, and direct communication; and generally what other aspects of the health care manager's leadership and style are most important to each subordinate. Moreover, it is important for the health care manager to know and understand their subordinates' employment and career goals, as these are considerations the health care manager must take into account in applying equity theory. Again, subordinates will take into account all these factors and others important to them as they assess how their treatment by the health care manager compares to coworkers and colleagues and whether they perceive it to be fair and equitable.

As it relates to assessing a health care workers' job readiness and psychological readiness, this requires the application of situational leadership theory, a leadership theory that states a manager should adjust their leadership style to the particular needs or aspects of their subordinates, placing importance on job readiness as well as psychological readiness to do the job. Job readiness has to do with the worker's knowledge, skills, abilities, competencies, and experience in doing the job or work. Psychological readiness has to do with the health care worker's motivation to do the job or work (Reed, 2018). For example, a registered nurse who has just graduated from nursing school at a university, but otherwise has no clinical nursing experience in the field, would probably need to be managed differently by the health care manager than a registered nurse with similar education but with 10 years of clinical experience working in direct patient care in a community hospital. All things being equal, the recent nursing graduate will need more supervision, training, coaching, and feedback than the nurse with 10 years of experience. In addition, two registered nurses with similar education and 10 years of similar clinical experience in a community hospital may have different levels of psychological readiness to do the job. One nurse may have much less motivation to do the work, and therefore will need more motivational leadership, which may include more attention, observation, coaching, feedback, and the like, in order to perform proficiently in the job. Situational leadership must be applied by health care leaders in a fair and equitable manner at all times.

A health care manager needs to be aware, make observations, seek feedback, and look for signs and clues, including subtle hints, ongoing as to their subordinates' perceptions of fairness and equitability with the manager's overall leadership and treatment of staff. Clearly there is a significant amount of emotional intelligence (EI, or EQ for emotional quotient) involved on the part of the health care manager as they monitor and assess subordinates' perception regarding the fairness and equitability of their treatment. Emotional intelligence can be defined as "*the capacity to be aware of, control, and express one's emotions, and to handle interpersonal relationships judiciously and empathetically*." (Oxford Languages, 2023). Another definition of EQ "*is the ability to perceive, interpret, demonstrate, control, evaluate, and use emotions to communicate with and relate to others effectively and constructively.* This ability to express and control emotions is essential, but so is the ability to understand, interpret, and respond to the emotions of others. Some experts suggest that Emotional Intelligence is more important than IQ for success in life" (Cherry, 2024).

This awareness should include not only what subordinates as well as coworkers and others may say, but also hints and clues as to what isn't said in certain situations. As Peter Drucker, considered the godfather of management, once said:

> "The most important thing in communication is to hear what isn't being said."
>
> ("Peter F. Drucker 1909–2005," n.d.)

Therefore, health care managers need to ensure they are fair and equitable in the treatment of their subordinates and teams by avoiding favoritism, giving workers equal opportunities to demonstrate their capabilities, and recognizing and rewarding workers fairly based upon effort, performance, and merit. Moreover, providing direct and appropriate feedback is important so subordinates clearly see and understand how their efforts, performance, and contributions compare to their colleagues and coworkers. Providing direct, clear, transparent communication to both subordinates individually and teams collectively is important to ensure health care workers are kept informed and understand how efforts, performance, and contributions are assessed by managers, and how they may be compared or benchmarked—internally or even externally.

LEADERSHIP ACTION STEPS FOR ADAMS'S EQUITY THEORY OF MOTIVATION

1. A health care manager should take the time and make the effort to get to know and understand subordinates well; this is time and effort well spent by the health care manager and can provide them with a foundation of knowledge and understanding in which they can effectively apply equity theory in their overall leadership.
2. A health care manager should ask subordinates directly, as well as look for hints and clues as to what aspects of their leadership, as well as the overall employment relationship, are most important to each subordinate. Moreover, the manager needs to inquire and pay attention to hints, clues, and other signs as to the subordinate's perceptions of their treatment and whether the subordinate feels it is fair and equitable, including in comparison to coworkers and others.
3. A health care manager needs to know and understand a subordinate's general psychological makeup, including job readiness and psychological readiness to do the job, as well as employment and career goals. A health care manager needs to understand the rationale and virtues of situational leadership, and how to apply it in a way that fosters a strong sense of fairness and equity for each subordinate.
4. A health care manager should always be clear and transparent with subordinates, as well as teams, and explain the ***why***—the reason or rationale for employment decisions as well as other operational decisions. While the health care manager can't share information that is private and confidential in nature, he should be clear about those aspects in his communication so subordinates will understand—and appreciate—those situations and considerations that are private and confidential.
5. A health care manager should provide direct, clear, specific, and appropriate feedback to subordinates and teams so they may see and understand how their efforts, performance, and contributions are being evaluated by management. Providing direct, clear, specific, and transparent communication to both subordinates individually and teams collectively is important to ensure health care workers are kept informed and understand how efforts, performance, and contributions

are assessed by managers and how they may be compared or benchmarked—internally or even externally.

6. Health care managers need to ensure they are fair and equitable in the treatment of their subordinates and teams by avoiding favoritism, giving health care workers equal opportunities to demonstrate their capabilities, and recognizing and rewarding health care workers fairly based upon effort, performance, and merit.
7. A health care manager needs to be aware, make observations, seek feedback, and look for signs, including subtle hints, ongoing as to subordinates' perceptions of fairness and equitability with the managers' overall leadership and treatment of staff. This awareness should include not only what subordinates as well as coworkers and others may say, but also hints and clues as to what isn't said in certain situations. Clearly there is a significant amount of emotional intelligence involved on the part of the health care manager as they monitor and assess subordinates' perception regarding the fairness and equitability of their treatment.

Assessing One's Leadership Style and Adams's Equity Theory of Motivation

The following questions are designed to prompt reflection and self-assessment, and to promote self-awareness and better understanding and insight about how you—as a student, health care manager, or leader—can use or are using Adams's equity theory of motivation with your own leadership style. Use the following 5-point Likert scale for this assessment:

5 = Always 4 = Sometimes 3 = Neutral 2 = Seldom 1 = Rarely/Never

1. I take the time and make the effort to get to know and understand each one of my subordinates and what is important to them, including career and employment goals, so that I can consistently and appropriately apply equity theory in my leadership.

   5 4 3 2 1

2. I routinely and consistently observe my subordinates doing the work and interact with them about the work they are doing and how they are performing, providing them with clear, direct, specific, and constructive feedback.

5 4 3 2 1

3. I routinely assess the knowledge, skills, abilities, competencies, and motivation of my subordinates and appropriately apply situational leadership in conjunction with equity theory in my leadership style.

5 4 3 2 1

4. I ask my subordinates directly, and routinely and consistently look for hints, clues, and signs as to what aspects of my leadership and their employment relationship are most important to my subordinates and their perceptions of fairness and equitability in their treatment.

5 4 3 2 1

- List two or three of the most frequent ways you look for hints, clues, and signs as to what aspects of your leadership and the employment relationship are most important to your subordinates and their perceptions of fairness and equitability in their treatment:
    - A.
    - B.
    - C.

5. I am always clear and transparent with subordinates with my communication and explain the ***why***—the reason or rationale for employment decisions as well as other operational decisions. I don't share private and confidential information, but I am clear about those aspects I can't share in my communication so subordinates will understand—and appreciate—those situations and considerations.

   5 4 3 2 1

6. While I make observations, seek feedback, and look for signs, clues, and subtle hints ongoing about my subordinate's perceptions of fairness and equitability with my overall leadership and treatment of staff, I am also *cognizant of what isn't being said* in certain situations, using my emotional intelligence to assess subordinate perceptions regarding fairness and equitability of their treatment.

   5 4 3 2 1

____

____

____

____

References

Cherry, K. (2024, January 31). Emotional intelligence: How we perceive, evaluate, express, and control emotions. Verywell Mind. https://www.verywellmind.com/what-is-emotional-intelligence-2795423

Davlembayeva, D., & Alamanos, E. (2023). Equity theory: A review. In S. Papagiannidis (Ed), *TheoryHub Book*. ISBN: 9781739604400. https://open.ncl.ac.uk/theories/5/equity-theory/

Mata, Á. N. de S., de Azevedo, K. P. M., Braga, L. P., de Medeiros, G. C. B. S., de Oliveira Segundo, V. H., Bezerra, I. N. M., Pimenta, I. D. S. F., Nicolás, I. M., & Piuvezam, G. (2021). Training in communication skills for self-efficacy of health professionals: A systematic review. *Human Resources for Health, 19*(1), 1–9.

Oxford Languages. (2023). Oxford Languages and Google - English -. Languages.oup.com. https://languages.oup.com/google-dictionary-en

"Peter F. Drucker 1909–2005." (n.d.) Oxford Reference. https://www.oxfordreference.com/display/10.1093/acref/9780191826719.001.0001/q-oro-ed4-00012211

Reed, S. B. (2018). *Becoming a healthcare leader.* Cognella Academic Publishing.
Skills Communication. (2021, February 3). https://www.skillscommunication.fr/2021/02/03https://link.springer.com/article/10.1186/s12960-021-00574-3.
World of Work. (2019, February). Adams' equity theory of motivation: A simple summary. https://worldofwork.io/2019/02/adams-equity-theory-of-motivation/

Creditlines

Fig. 9.1a: Source: https://worldofwork.io/2019/02/adams-equity-theory-of-motivation/.
Fig. 9.1b: Source: https://worldofwork.io/2019/02/adams-equity-theory-of-motivation/.

CHAPTER 10

Victor Vroom's Expectancy Theory of Motivation

When I think about times when my motivation to do something, complete something, or achieve something has been high, there were three different factors or criteria that were also strong for me: (a) I believed in my ability to put forth the type of effort that would lead to high performance; (b) I believed that my performance would then satisfactorily complete the job or achieve the desired goal or outcome; and (c) I believed the desired goal or outcome was something desirable and worth the effort. Think of a time when you were highly motivated to do something, complete something, or achieve something. Did you believe in your abilities to give the effort needed? Did you believe your effort would result in a level of performance that was needed or required? And did you believe the task that you wanted to complete or goal you wanted to achieve was desirable and worth the effort you would have to make? According to Victor Vroom, the answer to these three questions is *yes*.

However, sometimes our beliefs around these three questions may not be a resounding ***yes***. Sometimes our beliefs around these three questions may be better described *as, **I have to try—so I'll give it my best effort and we will see how things turn out***, or, ***I really can't fail at this, so I'll have to give it my best***. The point here is that you can be motivated by the fear of failing, or the desire to avoid a particular negative outcome as well.

Background and Overview

Victor Vroom is a Canadian-born business school professor at the Yale School of Management at the time of this writing. In addition, Vroom has been a consultant for a number of large companies that include the likes of GE and American Express. Vroom's primary research involved explanation as to why individuals choose to follow certain courses of action and prefer certain goals or outcomes over others in organizations, particularly as it relates to leadership and leadership decision-making. Vroom's most recognized books are *Work and Motivation, Leadership and Decision Making*, and *The New Leadership*. Vroom suggests that motivation is largely influenced by the combination of one's belief that effort leads to performance, which then in turn leads to specific outcomes, and that such outcomes are valued by the individual. Vroom described the valence of a specific outcome as follows: "The force on a person to perform an act is a monotonically increasing function of the algebraic sum of the products of the valences of all other outcomes and his conceptions of its instrumentality for the attainment of these other outcomes" (Vroom quoted in "Victor Vroom," 2024). Therefore, Vroom's theory suggests that motivation is dependent upon the strength or likelihood the act or behavior will generate or be followed by a certain outcome. In other words, motivation is the product or result of an individual's expectations, and that a certain amount of effort will result in the expected performance, a tool for such performance will yield certain results, and the desirability of the result for the individual is worthwhile.

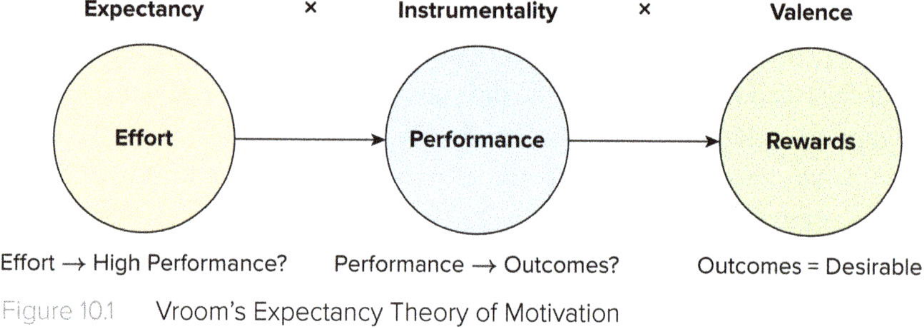

Figure 10.1 Vroom's Expectancy Theory of Motivation

Let's break down Vroom's expectancy theory of motivation into its three primary components. Expectancy is the measure of confidence the individual has in making the efforts needed to produce the desired performance. Expectancy involves the individual asking, *Will my effort lead to high performance*? Instrumentality is the measure of belief or confidence the employee has in the manager or organization delivering the rewards implied or promised. Instrumentality involves the employee asking, *Will my performance lead to the desired outcome*? Valence is the measure of value an individual attaches to a given outcome or reward, be it an intrinsic or extrinsic reward. Valence involves the employee asking, *Will the outcome or reward be worth the effort*? As a result, there is strong employee motivation when there is high expectancy, high instrumentality, and high valance at the same time. The theory is based upon the relationship between expectancy (effort), instrumentality (performance), and valence (reward), and the respective strength of each. When there are two of the criteria that are strong, but the third criteria is low or weak, it is believed there is moderate employee motivation at play. When two of the three criteria are low or weak, it is believed there is low motivation. When all three of the criteria are low or weak, it is believed there is strong avoidance (Papertyari, n.d.).

As defined in Chapter 3, situational leadership is a leadership theory or principle that suggests a subordinate should be managed by their supervisor as it relates to two factors: (a) the subordinate's job readiness, which refers to the knowledge, skills, and abilities to do the job, and (b) the subordinate's psychological readiness, which refers to the motivation to do the job (The Center for Leadership Studies, n.d.). As it relates to the expectancy theory of motivation, Vroom simplifies the combination of job readiness and psychological readiness by stating that:

> "Motivation depends on how much we want something and how likely we think we are to get it."
>
> (Pilat & Krastev, 2024).

Expectancy Theory Applies to Health Care Leaders, Workers, and Patients Alike

Expectancy theory applies to health care leaders, workers, and patients alike. The question *Will efforts lead to high performance and produce the outcomes desired?* applies to

1. health care leaders looking to motivate and inspire employees to work hard to achieve organizational goals; those same leaders using motivational techniques to drive higher levels of performance and outcomes on the part of health care workers; and leaders believing employee performance will lead to desirable outcomes;

2. motivated health care workers believing their efforts will lead to high performance; those same workers believing their performance will be on target to get the job done in a way that will produce outcomes; and the worker's believing their effort and performance will generate outcomes that are desired; and
3. patients believing their physician and team of caregivers will perform at a high level in terms of their patient care; those same patients believing all the tests, interventions, and caregiving they are receiving will result in clinical outcomes for the patient; and patients believing the clinical outcomes will lead to an improved health status in their condition.

As you read the above examples involving health care leaders, workers, and patients, you probably came to the conclusion there is a certain amount of trust involved with believing certain efforts will generate the type of performance which will lead to desired outcomes—which is true. Belief and trust are clearly part of this motivational theory and its application in practice.

Key Takeaways for Health Care Leaders

Organizational goals, department goals, and individual employee goals are important in a variety of ways, including the fact they should be designed or written to be motivating. This also applies to work tasks, assignments, and projects that are required to be done or completed on a daily basis. As we've discussed above, the three factors of effort, performance, and rewards may not all be highly motivating individually; however, collectively, these three factors need to be high or strong enough to provide the needed motivation for a health care worker's effort and performance to get the needed work done at a high level.

However, past practices and the organizational culture also play a significant role in employee motivation. Health care managers must always be cognizant of the following:

> Past precedent with regard to recognition and reward creates powerful inertia—that is, employee expectations for future recognition and reward.

While recognition and reward can certainly be changed and improved moving forward, past precedent sets an expectation with employees that future recognition and reward will be **at least** as good or attractive as what has occurred in the past.

The fear of failure can also be motivating. The fear of failure can include not wanting to look bad in the eyes of others; taking great pride in our work and not wanting others to perceive our work as less than adequate or less than our best; or failing to produce an outcome or achieve something that we have been asked to do, have volunteered to do, or that is just part of our job. The fear of failure can also include something like our fear of letting our team down when the team is reliant on our work or work product (which in health care is nearly 100% of the time). While the fear of failure can be motivating, health care managers are strongly discouraged—as a general rule—from using fear to motivate subordinates and teams. Motivating through fear is no longer suggested, advised, or much tolerated in our society today; it is not sustainable; and it has a high probability of backfiring or producing more negatives than positives. On the other hand, the fear of failure can be an inner drive that motivates a health care manager to give their discretionary effort and work hard to perform, contribute, and excel—which is fairly common. Therefore, the fear of failure isn't necessarily negative, as it can be an effective driver of motivation in the appropriate context within an individual health care manager. However, a word of caution here:

> Health care managers who use the fear of failure as a driver for their own internal motivation must be cognizant of this and careful not to lose perspective and let failures demotivate, demoralize, or create burnout.

Moreover, health care managers who use fear of failure as a driver for their own internal motivation must not allow this fear to become too intense, to result in loss of control, or to drive inappropriate thoughts, actions, or behaviors. Again, things must always be kept in perspective and we must learn from our mistakes, setbacks, and failures, and not dwell on them, beat ourselves up because of them, or become paranoid from them. As Henry Ford is believed to have said, "Failure is simply the opportunity to begin again, this time more intelligently." (IPL.org, 2021).

LEADERSHIP ACTION STEPS FOR THE EXPECTANCY THEORY OF MOTIVATION

1. **Know and understand your subordinates and teams, including their capabilities, wants, and desires**. In order to appropriately assign or delegate tasks, assignments, or projects effectively, a health care manager must know and understand the knowledge, skills, abilities, capabilities, potential, and psychological readiness/motivation to do the work of each of their subordinates and teams. Moreover, the health care manager must know and understand the wants and desires of subordinates and teams as well, in order to properly connect their effort, performance, and contributions to the appropriate recognition and reward (Indeed Editorial Team, 2024).
2. **Make sure your promises to subordinates and teams align with company goals and policies**. As a health care manager, promise keeping is crucial to maintaining believability, trust, and credibility. For example, in your current health care management position, do you have the authority to make the commitment you are contemplating to your subordinate? If you are contemplating paying a monetary bonus if certain goals or quantifiable targets are attained, do you have the authority to do so? Does company policy allow this or does corporate culture support this? If not—or if you are not sure—first secure the approval of your boss before ever mentioning anything to your subordinate about a possible commitment you want to make.
3. **Create challenging but achievable goals**. As a health care manager, it is your responsibility to know and fully understand the knowledge, skills, abilities, capabilities, and psychological readiness/motivation to do the job of each of your subordinates. This knowledge and understanding about each of your subordinates is necessary in order to assign tasks and delegate authority and accountability appropriately. This knowledge and understanding of subordinates is also critical for collaborating with them when setting goals, objectives, or even key performance indicators (KPIs). Clearly, subordinates and teams must be appropriately challenged in their work, but also asked to pursue

achievable goals, targets, and outcomes that are clearly aligned with company and department goals and priorities.

4. **Set clear connections between performance and recognition or reward**. It is important that expectations be well-communicated, well-known, and well-understood. Clear connections between a subordinate or team's performance and expected recognition or reward must be readily apparent, known, and clearly understood. Recognition and reward can be based on anything from verbal recognition for ongoing effort being displayed to monetary rewards for newly established quantifiable goals with set targets. Keep in mind: Past precedent with regard to recognition and reward creates powerful inertia—that is, employee expectations about future recognition and reward are usually as high or higher than past precedent.
5. **Recognition and reward must be fair and logical**. Recognition and reward should match the effort, performance, and significance of the outcomes or contributions made. Equity theory suggests that all subordinates and team members will evaluate and judge whether recognition and reward was congruent with effort, performance, and contribution.
6. **Recognition and reward must account for unforeseen or mitigating circumstances**. There are many, many moving parts in the operations of any hospital or health care organization, and things frequently change. Therefore, a health care manager must be prepared to provide recognition and reward that is commensurate with effort, performance, and contributions when things change midstream—prior to a specific goal or outcome being reached, including when organizational priorities, goals, and policies change. As a general rule, health care managers should always give the benefit of the doubt to subordinates and teams in this regard to avoid potential hard feelings, animosity, or a loss of motivation on the part of employees—especially when they had nothing to do with the changes, or unforeseen or mitigating circumstances.

Assessing One's Leadership Style and the Expectancy Theory of Motivation

The following questions are designed to prompt reflection and self-assessment, and to promote better understanding and insight about how you—as a student, health care manager, or leader—can use or are using the expectancy theory of motivation with your own leadership style. Use the following 5-point Likert scale for this assessment:

5 = Always 4 = Sometimes 3 = Neutral 2 = Seldom 1 = Rarely/Never

1. I know and understand the knowledge, skills, and abilities, as well as the job readiness, capabilities, potential, and expectations of my subordinates as well as teams.

   5 4 3 2 1

2. I know and understand the wants and desires of my subordinates and teams, and what forms of recognition and reward they find the most and the least important, meaningful, and motivating.

   5 4 3 2 1

3. I work individually with subordinates and collectively with my teams and department as a whole using participatory leadership to create challenging but achievable goals, objectives, and key performance indicators (KPIs) while setting clear expectations around the connections between performance and recognition and reward.

   5 4 3 2 1

- List two or three of the most frequent or effective ways you do this:
  A.
  B.
  C.

4. I am always cognizant and thoughtful about providing recognition and reward that is fair, logical, and matches the effort, performance, and significance of the outcomes or contributions made by subordinates and teams, appropriate with company culture, policy, past precedent, and equity theory.

   5 4 3 2 1

5. I accommodate for changes in priorities, goals, objectives, work assignments, policies, and staffing prior to a specific goal or outcome being reached, always giving the benefit of the doubt to subordinates and teams in this regard, appropriate with company culture, policy, and past precedent.

   5 4 3 2 1

____

____

____

____

References

The Center for Leadership Studies. (n.d.). *Situational leadership.* Retrieved July 10, 2024, from https://situational.com/situational-leadership/

Indeed Editorial Team. (2024, August 15). *8 Types of Employee Recognition (And Why It's Important).* Indeed Career Guide. https://www.indeed.com/career-advice/career-development/types-of-employee-recognition

Ipl.org. (2021, March 31). Essay On Failure Is Simply The Opportunity To Begin Again. Ipl.org. https://www.ipl.org/essay/Essay-On-Failure-Is-Simply-The-Opportunity-PKCCR-FQBGXPV

Papertyari. (n.d.). *Vroom expectancy theory of motivation.* Retrieved July 10, 2024, from https://papertyari.com/general-awareness/management/vroom-expectancy-theory-motivation/

Pilat, D., & Krastev, Dr. S. (2024). Expectancy Theory. The Decision Lab. https://thedecisionlab.com/reference-guide/psychology/expectancy-theory

Victor Vroom. (n.d.). In Wikipedia. Retrieved July 10, 2024, from https://en.wikipedia.org/wiki/Victor_Vroom

Creditlines

Fig. 10.1: Source: https://papertyari.com/general-awareness/management/vroom-expectancy-theory-motivation/.

CHAPTER 11

Peter F. Drucker's Management by Objectives Process for Motivation

How do health care managers go about providing alignment between the work done by health care workers and the organization's mission, vision, established priorities, goals, and objectives? How can health care managers help provide a strong sense of commitment, purpose, satisfaction and accomplishment, motivation, and value on the part of health care workers for the work they do every day? How can health care workers use the participatory leadership process in a way that heightens their sense of contribution towards the organization's mission, and a sense of emotional ownership for their work and that of their organization? One way is by using management by objectives, or MBO.

Background and Overview

MBO is a methodology for health care managers to implement goal setting theory at the individual employee level. MBO was first developed by Peter F. Drucker and highlighted in his 1954 book, titled *The Practice of Management*. Drucker was one of the most well-known and influential thinkers on management, and his work continues to be used by managers worldwide. Drucker was among the first to depict management as a distinct function and responsibility. Drucker had five guiding principles for managing effectively: (a) setting objectives, (b) organizing the group (or team), (c) motivating and communicating, (d) measuring performance, and (e) developing people.

MBO was one of the many concepts and methods regarding effective management promulgated by Drucker. MBO is a management philosophy, as well as a system and four-step process in which the manager works with subordinates individually to develop objectives each subordinate will work towards completing or achieving over a designated time period. The objectives developed and pursued by each employee should be in alignment with the company's mission, vision, strategy, designated priorities, goals, and objectives. Here is the basic four-step MBO process:

1. Manager and subordinate meet to discuss possible objectives the subordinate might adopt.
2. Manager and subordinate agree upon the objectives the subordinate will pursue.
3. Manager and subordinate establish a regular interval or schedule for meeting to discuss progress being made by subordinate towards attaining objectives.
4. Manager and subordinate meet periodically to review and discuss subordinate's progress towards attaining objectives with appropriate manager support and feedback provided.

One of the central premises of the MBO process is the use of *participatory leadership*, whereby the health care manager engages and involves health care workers in the development of the objectives they will pursue. This collaboration between health care manager and health care worker helps the worker to feel more involved, more appreciated, more valuable, and subsequently more motivated to contribute effort and performance to the achievement and success of each objective. It is the participatory leadership process and providing the health care worker with opportunity for input into the development of objectives and collaboration with the health care manager that is pivotal in this process. As a result, health care workers are much more apt to have a higher level of motivation, commitment, and emotional ownership for working hard to achieve each objective they adopt. Drucker valued employee motivation, commitment, and emotional ownership for working hard:

> "Do not measure your life by your goals but what you are doing to achieve them."
>
> (Abbate, 2020)

Drucker also believed in keeping the number of goals or objectives that an individual had at any one time to only a few:

> “If you have more than five goals, you have none.”
>
> (Sprague, 2019)

While MBO was promulgated in the mid-20th century, there are a number of large, notable companies that still use MBO today, including Hewlett-Packard, Xerox, and Intel (Levinson, 2014). Research published in December 2021 from the International Conference on Decision Aid Sciences and Application, titled “*The Impact of Management by Objectives on Employee Behaviour and Performance*,” showed findings that the use of MBO creates a state of employee motivation, satisfaction, commitment, and loyalty (George et al., 2021).

MBO Can Be Used in Health Care Worker Performance Appraisal and Evaluation

While MBO can help facilitate health care worker effort and performance in a desired direction, it can also prove to be an important component when appraising or evaluating a health care worker’s performance. When a health care leader works collaboratively with a health care worker to establish objectives the health care worker will work to achieve, the established objectives can (and should) also be used, at least in part, to evaluate and assess the health care worker’s efforts and performance during a given period, such as a performance appraisal period. Written objectives that both the health care leader and worker have discussed, agreed upon, and have worked towards achieving should be a component of what the worker’s efforts and performance are evaluated on. By doing so, the health care worker will feel this component of their performance appraisal is based upon objectives that are known, clear, specific to the employee, and understood by both the health care leader and worker. Moreover, this approach provides the health care worker with input into what their performance will be evaluated on, providing a greater sense of commitment, buy-in, and support, and overall satisfaction from the worker, while helping to streamline or make efficient at least part of the performance appraisal process.

Key Takeaways for Health Care Leaders

MBO is a collaborative process between the health care manager and worker. Many times health care managers will need training in important areas where the manager must perform well in order to guide or coach the health care worker, such as how to develop SMART goals; how to create goal alignment between individual health care worker objectives and organizational goals; how to work collaboratively with subordinates in developing their objectives; how to monitor progress towards achievement of objectives and provide appropriate feedback; and how to evaluate success using achievement of objectives as part of the subordinate's overall performance appraisal process.

In addition to these key points, health care managers can initiate the MBO process in advance or in conjunction with the organization's key business cycles, such as budgeting, strategic planning, or even the health care worker's performance appraisal period. Using a health care workers' objectives as an important component for overall performance evaluation and appraisal is warranted, as it provides a clear and objective way to measure and evaluate a subordinate's efforts and performance for a specific time period for each specific objective the health care manager and worker have discussed, agreed to, and worked collaboratively to achieve.

As will be further discussed in Chapter 14 on the goal-setting theory of motivation, setting and accomplishing objectives through the MBO process can help foster a sense of purpose, satisfaction, and accomplishment for employees. Moreover, there is a direct connection between goal setting and workplace performance.

Setting goals and objectives can help

- clarify and visualize success;
- clarify purpose, priority, and direction for work to be performed;
- add recognizable value to the work an employee, a team, or an organization is doing;
- provide criteria to monitor and assess progress being made, and to recognize effort and performance towards goal achievement;
- create tactics for operational or performance efficiencies and improvements, as well as time management of tasks and workflow;
- motivate and increase energy, enthusiasm, effort, and performance in doing the work; and
- enhance teamwork and collaboration.

(Bard College Center for Civic Engagement, n.d.)

LEADERSHIP ACTION STEPS FOR MANAGEMENT BY OBJECTIVES

1. The health care manager should identify, review, understand, and discuss the organization's mission, vision, designated priorities, strategies, goals, and objectives with the subordinate to help establish overall direction and framework for discussions regarding possible objectives for the subordinate.
2. The health care manager and subordinate meet—multiple times as necessary—to discuss possible objectives that might be adopted by the subordinate.
3. The health care manager and subordinate meet to discuss and agree upon objectives that will be adopted by the subordinate, as well as the target time period for attainment. During this discussion the health care manager and subordinate should discuss what resources and support the subordinate will need in order to achieve the objectives, including any needed training or coaching. In addition, the health care manager should consider how best they might employ the Pygmalion effect in these discussions. (See Robert Rosenthal's Pygmalion effect for more detail on this topic.)
4. During the above meeting, or at a separate meeting, the health care manager and subordinate should discuss and agree upon a regular schedule of future meetings to discuss progress being made towards attainment of objectives, and any modifications, changes, or adjustments indicated, or additional support or resources the subordinate might need.
5. The health care manager and subordinate meet as agreed to discuss progress being made towards attainment of objectives, and any modifications, changes, or adjustments indicated, or additional support or resources the subordinate might need. The health care manager should provide feedback regarding the subordinate's efforts and performance, being mindful of things such as the expectancy theory of motivation and equity theory. The health care manager needs to be cognizant of how they might assist and support the subordinate towards attainment of the objectives at all times.

Assessing One's Leadership Style and Management by Objectives

The following questions are designed to prompt reflection and self-assessment, and to promote better understanding and insight about how you—as a student, health care manager, or leader—can use or are using management by objectives with your own leadership style. Use the following 5-point Likert scale for this assessment:

5 = Always 4 = Sometimes 3 = Neutral 2 = Seldom 1 = Rarely/Never

1. I routinely and consistently discuss important organizational, departmental, and individual objectives specific to each of my subordinates.

   5 4 3 2 1

2. I routinely and consistently work with my subordinates to establish individual objectives they agree to pursue for a designated time period, making sure each objective is in alignment with departmental and organization goals.

   5 4 3 2 1

3. I meet regularly with each subordinate individually to discuss progress being made toward attainment of each of their objectives, inquiring what additional support they may need and how I might assist in that regard, while providing the support needed whenever possible.

   5 4 3 2 1

4. I routinely and consistently provide feedback, encouragement, and reinforcement as appropriate to each subordinate as it relates to their efforts to achieve their objectives.

   5 4 3 2 1

- List up to three of the most frequent ways you do this:
  A.
  B.
  C.

5. I communicate with subordinates in appropriate ways as to how their efforts towards achieving their objectives help to achieve departmental and organizational goals, as well as the organization's mission.

5 4 3 2 1

___

___

___

___

References

Abbate, B. (2020, June 29). How to Apply Some of the Best Business Principles to Your Life. Medium; ILLUMINATION. https://medium.com/illumination/how-to-apply-some-of-the-best-business-principles-to-your-life-386df32c0641

Bard College Center for Civic Engagement. (n.d.). *Setting goals and objectives.* Retrieved July 10, 2024, from https://cce.bard.edu/files/Setting-Goals.pdf

Drucker, P. F. (1954). *The practice of management.* Harper & Brothers.

George, S., Al Jaber, M. K., Salem, M. J., & AlSaad, A. J. (2021). The impact of management by objectives on employee behaviour and performance. 2021 International Conference on Decision Aid Sciences and Application (DASA), Sakheer, Bahrain. https://doi.org/10.1109/DASA53625.2021.9682364

Levinson, H. (2014, August). Management by Whose Objectives? Harvard Business Review. https://hbr.org/2003/01/management-by-whose-objectives

Sprague, K. (2019, October 19). 21 Productivity Quotes from Peter Drucker That Are Perfect for Ambitious Millennials. Medium.com; Medium. https://karlwsprague.medium.com/21-productivity-quotes-from-peter-drucker-that-are-perfect-for-ambitious-millennials-ecabac9a967e

CHAPTER 12

Fred Edward Fiedler's Contingency Theory of Leadership

Once a health care manager develops an effective leadership style, does that mean their leadership style should be applied the same to all subordinates? In all situations? Fred Edward Fiedler's answer to this question would be a resounding no! A health care manager must develop their own leadership style based on their personality, personal characteristics and traits, values, beliefs, education, training, and experience. However, how a health care manager applies their leadership style is another matter altogether, and one that Fiedler suggests depends on the situation or circumstances.

Fiedler's contingency theory is grounded in the premise that certain leaders—based upon their natural leadership style, which he believed was basically fixed and inflexible—would be appropriate and effective for certain situations or circumstances where there is a match (Mind Tools, n.d.). However, this approach is based on the belief that leaders can't flex or change their leadership style to match the situation or circumstances. My experience tells me otherwise. My experience tells me that a leader can and should flex their approach or leadership style to match the situation or circumstances. In what is also called situational leadership, a leader can alter their leadership style to match the employee's psychological readiness (motivation to do the work) and job readiness (knowledge, skills, abilities, and experience) (The Center for Leadership Studies, n.d.).

For example, it seems straightforward that a nursing care manager would lead/manage/supervise a recent nursing graduate right out of a BSN nursing program differently than they would a registered nurse with 10 years or more of experience in nursing and who has worked on the same nursing service or unit in the same hospital for her entire career. In general, a recent nursing graduate will need more on-the-job training, coaching, direction, and supervision than the registered nurse with over 10 years of experience—at least in the beginning. In addition, the recent nursing graduate may need more feedback, positive encouragement, positive reinforcement, and overall support than the experienced nurse. As it relates to the Hawthorne effect, the recent graduate may need to have her direct supervisor a bit more visible and accessible in the beginning as well.

Fiedler's contingency theory of leadership isn't a motivational theory per se; however, it is important as it relates to a leader's ability to motivate and inspire subordinates, as well as those around them, by using an appropriate and effective leadership style, given the specific situation or circumstances.

> "The quality of leadership, more than any other single factor, determines the success or failure of an organization."
>
> (Fiedler quoted in van Vliet, 2024)

Background and Overview

Fred Edward Fiedler was an Austrian-born psychologist, emeritus professor, and one of the leading researchers of industrial and organizational psychology and organizational performance in the 20th century. Fiedler was 15 years old when his country was invaded by Hitler's German army and he and his family fled Austria, ending up in South Bend, Indiana.

Fiedler's contingency theory of leadership recognizes that there are many factors and variables that influence leadership behavior and effectiveness as well as organizational effectiveness, and that different leadership actions and behaviors are required for different situations and circumstances. In addition, Fiedler suggests that organizational structures must fit and support leadership styles in order for overall performance to be enhanced. One significant factor that should otherwise be noted with the contingency equation is the organization's culture and role it plays as well—particularly as it relates to Fiedler's reference to organizational structures.

Fiedler studied various areas of activity in the field of effective leadership. Years of study lead to his groundbreaking book, *Theory of Leadership Effectiveness*, published in 1967. In his book, Fiedler identified how leadership effectiveness and organizational performance are directly linked, and that leadership effectiveness is dependent upon the leader's actions and behaviors as they relate to the organizational situation and circumstances. Over the years, Fiedler's work has been published in numerous books and articles, starting with his book *Leader Attitudes and Group Effectiveness* in 1958, up until his last publication in 1994, *Leadership Experience and Leadership Performance* (van Vliet, 2024).

Fiedler's contingency theory suggests that effective leadership is contingent upon a match between the leader's style and the situational demands the leader faces in their position, organizational culture, and internal environment. In other words, a one-size-fits-all leadership style just won't be effective.

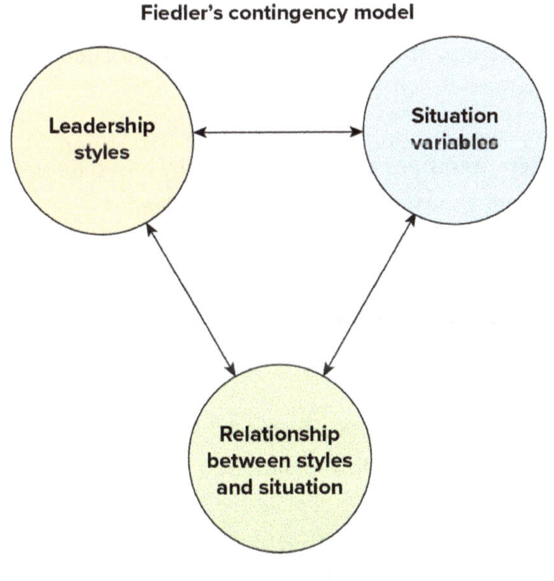

Figure 12.1 Fiedler's Contingency Model

Fiedler's theory suggests that a health care manager should be selected for the position or task at hand based upon their natural leadership style and what the situation or circumstances dictate is needed. As noted above, Fiedler's contingency theory is grounded in the premise that certain leaders—depending upon their natural leadership style, which he believed was basically fixed and inflexible—would be appropriate and effective for certain situations or circumstances where there is a match (between the leader's style of leadership and the style of leadership warranted by the situation or circumstances).

Fiedler developed a model called the Least-Preferred Coworker (LPC) scale as a way to measure leadership style. The LPC scale featured a table with sixteen personality traits or characteristics and a rating scale from 1 to 8. Personality traits or characteristics used in the LPC scale included unfriendly/friendly, cold/warm, rejecting/accepting, backbiting/loyal, unkind/kind and untrustworthy/trustworthy. The LPC scale suggests that task-oriented leaders view their LPCs more negatively, resulting in lower scores, while relationship-oriented leaders usually view their LPCs more positively, resulting in higher scores. The LPC scale was a way to identify whether the leader was basically a relationship-oriented leader, or a task-oriented leader.

Next, to apply the Fiedler contingency model, one determines the situational favorableness of the particular situation or circumstances with the leader's style using three distinct factors:

1. **Leader–member relations,** principally based upon the trust and confidence the employees have in the leader
2. **Task structure** or the degree the tasks are clear, structured, and achievable
3. **Leader's position power** or amount of authority the leader has to direct and control the team, including to reward or punish

Again, as mentioned above, the model attempts to provide for a match between the leader's style and the situation or circumstances (Mind Tools, n.d.).

Health Care Leaders Typically Hired Based Upon Their Leadership Philosophy and Style

Typically, a health care leader is hired because of their leadership philosophy and style. In most hiring situations, one or more potential candidates are interviewed for a given health care leadership position and evaluated, based in large part on the leadership philosophy and style the candidate espouses and portrays to the those doing the interviewing. Clearly, in most hiring situations there are other criteria used to evaluate a candidate's appropriateness and fit for a given health care leadership position than just their leadership philosophy and style; however, leadership philosophy and style are typically front and center, and considered more important than most other hiring criteria. Therefore, in general, most health care organizations use the philosophy and thinking behind Fidler's contingency model in their respective hiring processes. Health care organizations are typically trying to find the right fit in leadership philosophy and style given the particular situation and circumstances of the health care leadership position being filled.

However, according to situational leadership, a health care leader must flex or adjust their leadership style to fit the situation and circumstances involved with a leadership position, including the psychological readiness and job readiness of the employees (The Center for Leadership Studies, n.d.). In other words, while a health care leader's natural leadership philosophy will guide his or her leadership style in action; and different leadership philosophies and styles may be more or less appropriate for a given health care leadership position; a health care leader must always be cognizant of a health care leadership position's situation and circumstances, along with the psychological readiness and job readiness of the health care workers.

Key Takeaways for Health Care Leaders

A leader must be self-aware of his natural leadership style. In large part, a leader's own natural leadership style will likely be based upon his personality and related personal attributes, characteristics, values and beliefs. What makes this both complicated and challenging is that a leader's natural leadership style has many, many dimensions. One method a leader can use to assess his leadership style is through self-reflection. Self-reflection involves identifying and assessing situations and circumstances with subordinates or even colleagues or coworkers that have already occurred where the health care manager has provided leadership. What did the health care manager do well? How did others accept or react to the health care manager's words, actions or behaviors and what can be learned? What could the health care manager improve? Upon reflection, what steps should the health care manager take to improve his leadership effectiveness in the future, both regarding interpersonal relations as well as task-oriented actions?

Another method to assess one's leadership style includes informally soliciting feedback and insight from trusted/respected colleagues, a coach or mentor, or even supervisor. A related method that can provide helpful insight is through the use of the 360-degree evaluation process where a leadership evaluation tool is completed by the leader, 3 to 5 subordinates, 3 to 5 peers, and the leader's direct supervisor—all responding to the same questionnaire as to the various attributes, tendencies and traits commonly displayed by the leader in action. Using this 360-degree evaluation method, the leader can compare perceptions and insights about his leadership from those he leads, his colleagues and peers, and his supervisor to that of his own self-perception of his leadership style, which will typically highlight gaps and different perceptions held by others that may need to be addressed by the leader.

Another method that can be used to provide a leader with insight into his leadership style is by taking a personality profile test such as Myers-Briggs or DISC. Personality profile testing can provide a leader (or anyone) with insight into how they naturally work, think, and act and therefore might be perceived by others, or related to by others in a workplace or leadership setting. A point to note here is that each personality profile test available today has its own benefits and drawbacks; therefore, it may be wise to not rely solely on one but a combination of at least two or more different personality profile tests.

Health care managers who are effective at applying Situational Leadership are those who are able to flex or alter their leadership style or approach given the health care worker, health care team, organizational culture, situation or circumstance at hand (The Center for Leadership Studies, n.d.). In the example previously given regarding the new graduate nurse versus the experienced registered nurse, the new graduate will most likely need more encouragement, support, and coaching—at least in the beginning. Can the health care manager provide encouragement, support, and coaching in the appropriate amount and ways that will be most effective for the new graduate? Moreover, does the health care manager have the emotional intelligence to know and understand what the most appropriate amount and ways are to provide encouragement, support, and coaching for this health care worker? The ability to know and understand what methods, approaches, and techniques might work best for a given health care worker, plus the ability to apply and use those methods, approaches, and techniques when appropriate is a big part of effectively applying situational leadership with the effective use of emotional intelligence.

LEADERSHIP ACTION STEPS FOR FIEDLER'S CONTINGENCY THEORY

1. Work to understand situational leadership and when and how it can best be applied in health care leadership settings and circumstances with the use of emotional intelligence.
2. Are you more task-oriented or more relationship-oriented overall? Use one or more means as noted above to better understand your own personality and natural leadership style, which includes your own personality profile and natural predilections towards work, stress, frustration, challenges, task completion, and interactions with others.
3. Work on improving your emotional intelligence and self-awareness, particularly in the early stages of your health care career. Assess your own natural tendencies—especially in different environments, situations, or circumstances, or with different people or groups. Identify how you typically show up in these environments, and what triggers prompt you towards certain emotions, feelings, or behaviors. Develop indicators and techniques that help you identify your emotions and feelings in their very early stages and manage or control them to help you be more consistent, appropriate, and professional in your actions and behaviors. Emotional intelligence also includes your ability to assess how others perceive or respond to you or different situations or circumstances.
4. Develop your leadership philosophy and leadership style to include multiple different methods, approaches, and techniques that you can apply appropriately given the subordinate, the team, the organizational culture, and the situation or circumstances. For example, learn how best to be a more relationship-oriented leader or a more task-oriented leader depending on what is appropriate for the subordinate, the team, the organizational culture, and the situation or circumstances at any given moment.

5. Be cognizant—at all times—of both when and how to flex or alter your leadership style, depending upon the subordinate, the team, the organizational culture, and the situation or circumstances. This includes knowing when and how much, or to what degree, to flex or alter your leadership style, including when and how to make changes and adjustments ongoing, given what is most needed.

Assessing One's Leadership Style and Fiedler's Contingency Theory

The following questions are designed to prompt reflection and self-assessment, and to promote better understanding and insight about how you—as a student, health care manager, or leader—can use or are using Fiedler's contingency theory with your own leadership style. Use the following 5-point Likert scale for this assessment:

5 = Always 4 = Sometimes 3 = Neutral 2 = Seldom 1 = Rarely/Never

1. I know and understand situational leadership and when, and how, and to what degree to best apply it with various health care workers as well as leadership settings and circumstances.

   5 4 3 2 1

2. I know whether I am more task-oriented or more relationship-oriented in my natural leadership style. I've used multiple methods to better understand my own natural leadership style, which includes my own personality profile and natural tendencies towards work, stress, frustration, challenges, task completion, and interactions with others.

   5 4 3 2 1

3. I have worked significantly to improve my emotional intelligence and self-awareness. I understand how I typically show up in different social and work environments, and what triggers prompt me towards certain feelings or behaviors, and have developed indicators and techniques that help me identify my emotions and feelings in their very early stages and manage or control them, resulting in consistent, appropriate, and professional behavior at all times. My aptitude with emotional intelligence (EI/EQ) also includes my ability to assess how others perceive or respond to me or different situations or circumstances, and I am accurate at predicting same.

   5 4 3 2 1

- List two or three of the most frequent ways you have worked to successfully improve your EI/EQ:
   A.
   B.
   C.

4. I have, and continue, to develop my leadership philosophy and leadership style to include multiple different methods, approaches, and techniques (including being more relationship-oriented or task-oriented as needed) that I can apply appropriately given the subordinate, the team, the organizational culture, and the situation or circumstances.

   5 4 3 2 1

5. I am cognizant—at all times—of both when and how to flex or alter my leadership style, depending upon the subordinate, the team, the organizational culture, and the situation or circumstances. In addition, I know when and how much, or to what degree, to flex or alter my leadership style, including when and how to make changes and adjustments ongoing, given what is most needed and appropriate.

   5 4 3 2 1

References

Fiedler, F. E. (1964). A contingency model of leadership effectiveness. *Advances in Experimental Social Psychology*, *1*, 149-190.

Mind Tools. (n.d.). *Fiedler's contingency model.* Retrieved July 10, 2024, from https://www.mindtools.com/ayfk2dg/fiedlers-contingency-model

The Center for Leadership Studies. (n.d.). *Situational leadership.* Retrieved July 10, 2024, from https://situational.com/situational-leadership/

van Vliet, V. (2024, May 28). *Fred Fiedler biography and leadership theory. Toolshero.* Retrieved July 10, 2024, from https://www.toolshero.com/toolsheroes/fred-fiedler/

Creditlines

Fig. 12.1: Source: https://www.quora.com/What-is-Fiedlers-contingency-theory-of-leadership.

CHAPTER 13

Robert Rosenthal's Pygmalion Effect

We show up every day with expectations about what we want to do, see, work on, accomplish, achieve, complete, start, and even think or write about. Sometimes our expectations for the day are about visiting, seeing, or being with a loved one, family member, or friend. Sometimes our expectations for the day are about going sightseeing, doing something we've never done before for fun, or enjoying a vacation. Sometimes our expectations for the day are about relaxing and taking things easy. Whatever our expectations, we have them: Sometimes our expectations are a bit cloudy and sometimes our expectations are clear and specific. Whatever the case, our expectations guide and structure our actions and motivations. In general, the greater and clearer our expectations are for achievement or accomplishment, and the more important or meaningful those expectations are to us, the greater effort we will give towards meeting those expectations. Furthermore, when others have high expectations for us that we support or subscribe to, and believe are achievable and important, we tend to elevate our efforts and performance to achieve those expectations. This reaction to higher expectations that others may have for us is called the Pygmalion effect.

Background and Overview

Robert Rosenthal, PhD, was a German-born American clinical psychologist who conducted research in both everyday life and in laboratory situations for over 50 years on the role of self-fulfilling prophecies. In 1964, Rosenthal conducted empirical research that set the stage for identification of the motivational concept called the Pygmalion effect, also called the Rosenthal effect, which involves the idea that expectations can bring about self-fulfilling prophecies. It is a theory showing that people will often end up behaving in the way that others had expected them to when the person has been repeatedly exposed to others' expectations about them. This effect can be both positive and negative in nature.

In Rosenthal's classic research study, elementary school teachers were told that, on the basis of psychological tests, some of their students were designated as either intellectual bloomers or late bloomers. Furthermore, even though they hadn't shown any academic success, those late bloomers were expected to bloom and show an intellectual growth spurt during the school year. In actuality, the students were randomly given the designation of intellectual bloomers. In a very short time, those teachers began to treat those children differently; those children began to think of themselves differently; and as a result, those children performed significantly better than the other students. In essence, these students were transformed by their teacher's positive expectations. Why? Because the teachers believed in the students, and unconsciously gave more positive attention, feedback, and learning opportunities to these students, which was viewed as teachers providing nonverbal communication of their positive expectations for the students and their academic success (Robert Rosenthal, 2009).

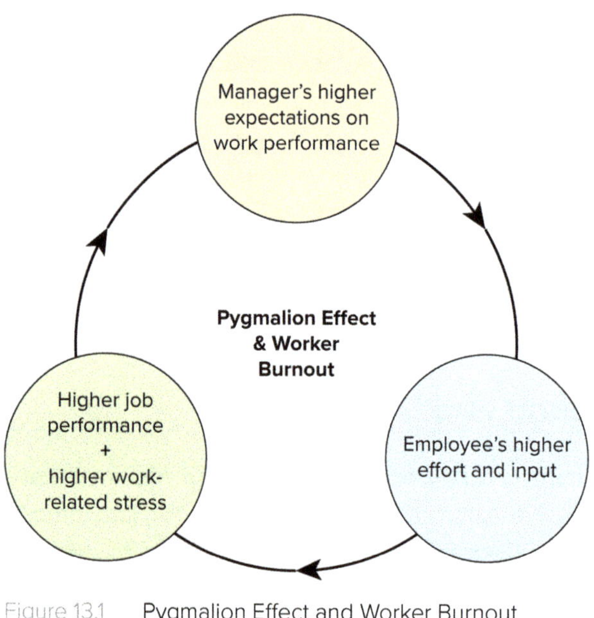

Figure 13.1 Pygmalion Effect and Worker Burnout

The power of the Pygmalion effect, first captured by Rosenthal in his study of elementary school children and their teachers, has been well documented as a simple and effective way to boost performance in the classroom, the workplace, the military, and in health care. The Pygmalion effect has been documented to improve employee performance, as published in an article titled "Pygmalion Leadership: The Power of Positive Expectations" (Riggio, 2009). In this article, author Ronald E. Riggio suggests that "*as a leader, simply holding positive expectations about team members' performance can actually lead to better team performance.*" Riggio goes on to state that "*we get the outcomes that we expect.*" Moreover, there was a meta-analysis completed which found that when leadership is trained to use the Pygmalion effect, it is a very effective leadership development intervention. The Pygmalion effect is named after George Bernard Shaw's play, in which Professor Henry Higgins transforms a common flower seller, Eliza Doolittle, into a lady because he believed that it would happen. (You likely are more familiar with the musical version, My Fair Lady.)

Health Care Leaders Can Inspire Workers by Setting and Conveying Realistic but High Expectations

A health care leader can apply the Pygmalion effect using many different techniques: Here is one. Let's assume a health care leader has evaluated and assessed one of their health care workers who has been doing a good job, but has the talent, skills, and abilities to perform at a much higher level than the worker has heretofore exhibited. The health care leader could then meet individually with the worker, in private, to discuss the worker's talents, skills, abilities, and performance potential. During this meeting, the health care leader can specifically describe expectations higher than those the worker is currently meeting, that the health care leader believes are reasonable and attainable for the worker. The Pygmalion effect suggests that the health care leader setting and conveying these higher expectations to the health care worker will motivate the worker to aspire and work towards those expectations, with one caveat: The health care worker must believe the expectations to be realistic and achievable. Therefore, it is the health care leader's job to be able to clearly articulate the higher expectations and support for the worker in a manner that is authentic, believable, and convincing. Moreover, a good dose of encouragement from the health care leader is also in order here.

Key Takeaways for Health Care Leaders

> *"As a leader, simply holding positive expectations about team members' performance can actually lead to better team performance. ... We get the outcomes that we expect."*
>
> *(Riggio, 2009)*

One of the primary takeaways from the Pygmalion effect is for health care managers to be mindful of the role both their communicated and implied expectations have on the effort and performance of subordinates and teams. Health care managers need to be sure their expectations of subordinates and teams are clear, realistic, achievable, and appropriate, and require the employee or team to display a high level of effort and performance to meet those expectations. The health care manager also needs to be sure expectations are made clear to employees and are well understood. It is also the health care manager's responsibility to be sure subordinates—or the team—have the resources and support needed to achieve the desired expectations, as well as exercise the basic management function of control in the process when appropriate, *monitoring progress towards goal achievement and taking any corrective action as necessary.*

Health care managers need know and understand what their subordinates and teams are capable of achieving, and what their potential for effort and performance is. This knowledge and understanding of a subordinate's capabilities is vital vis-à-vis the health care manager setting high but achievable performance expectations with their subordinates and teams. A health care manager needs to hold high expectations for subordinates and teams that are achievable, realistic, and meaningful. When a health care manager has high expectations that are realistic, achievable, and meaningful for subordinates, it can be motivating. As the Pygmalion effect suggests, higher expectations can provide the motivation for greater individual and team effort and performance.

While we have explored why a health care manager should focus on the Pygmalion effect when setting or communicating expectations for subordinates and teams, the Pygmalion effect also has application for health care managers themselves. What expectations do you, as a health care manager or aspiring health care manager, have for yourself, for your leadership, or for your effort and performance on a daily basis? As a health care manager, be sure you are thinking about and setting high expectations for yourself that are realistic, achievable, and appropriate, and that will require you to display a high level of effort and performance to meet those expectations. Health care managers are always being watched by their subordinates and others, and it is important for managers to model the way in terms of their own effort and performance, as an example for what they want to see from their subordinates. A manager's own expectations for themselves include things like having written agendas prepared and organized in advance of meetings and being prepared to speak; being to work on time and staying until the workday is through; providing ongoing and transparent communication to subordinates and teams, keeping them informed and updated; and modeling the way regarding adherence to policies and procedures and displaying a strong work ethic and performance. Managers are always modeling the way; they need to make sure what they are modeling for employees is what they expect from them.

LEADERSHIP ACTION STEPS FOR THE PYGMALION EFFECT

1. Health care managers need to set high expectations for subordinate and team performance that are achievable, realistic, and meaningful, based upon clear, open, and forthright communication and other actions and behaviors. Health care managers should not assume their subordinates, teams, and other coworkers or colleagues know what the manager's expectations are. Expectations for subordinates and teams should be discussed frequently and ongoing in the scheme of daily supervision and management of operations.
2. Health care managers need to ask their subordinates, coworkers, colleagues, and others as appropriate about their own expectations for their individual work effort and performance, and not assume they know.
3. Expectations need to be discussed frequently and clarified to be sure all are aware and understand, especially when there are new organizational or departmental strategies, goals, priorities, policies,

procedures, tasks, positions, job assignments, projects, workflow, staffing schedules, and the like.

4. Health care managers should discuss individual expectations with subordinates during performance evaluation sessions, management by objectives (MBO) sessions, or discussions about opportunities or possibilities for advancements or promotions. Health care managers should have high expectations for subordinates that are achievable, realistic, and meaningful. At the same time, these discussions should include some comparison of each person's respective expectations regarding same.
5. Managers need to understand the knowledge, skills, abilities, and competencies of each subordinate and what their performance potential and overall capabilities are. This knowledge and understanding is critical for the manager to work collaboratively with subordinates in the MBO process, as is having and discussing high expectations regarding effort, performance, and contributions that are realistic and achievable.

Assessing One's Leadership Style and the Pygmalion Effect

The following questions are designed to prompt reflection and self-assessment, and to promote better understanding and insight about how you—as a student, health care manager, or leader—can use or are using the Pygmalion effect with your own leadership style. Use the following 5-point Likert scale for this assessment:

5 = Always 4 = Sometimes 3 = Neutral 2 = Seldom 1 = Rarely/Never

1. I routinely and consistently communicate my high expectations for work efforts and performance to my subordinates, coworkers, colleagues, and teams in clear, open, and forthright terms ongoing in the scheme of daily supervision and operations, and don't assume employees know what those expectations are.

   5 4 3 2 1

- List two or three of the most frequent ways you do this, and/or forums or environments you do this in:
    A.
    B.
    C.

2. I routinely and consistently ask my subordinates, coworkers, colleagues, and teams, as appropriate, about their own expectations for their work efforts and performance, and don't assume I know what these expectations are.

    5 4 3 2 1

3. I routinely and consistently include expectations when discussing strategies, goals, objectives, key performance indicators, new committees or teams, new priorities, policies and procedures, tasks, positions, job assignments, projects, workflow, staffing schedules, and the like.

    5 4 3 2 1

4. I routinely and consistently discuss individual expectations with subordinates during performance evaluation sessions, management by objectives sessions, opportunities or possibilities for advancements or promotions, and so on, comparing the subordinate's own expectations regarding the same.

    5 4 3 2 1

5. I work hard to understand the knowledge, skills, abilities, and competencies of each subordinate and what their performance potential and overall capabilities are in order to work collaboratively in the MBO process, as well as discuss and establish high expectations regarding effort, performance, contributions, and so on.

    5 4 3 2 1

References

Panmore Institute. (n.d.). *Pygmalion effect.* Retrieved July 10, 2024, from https://www.google.com/search?rlz=1C1GCEB_enUS917US917&q=pygmalion+effect&tbm=isch&sa=X&ved=2ahUKEwjt0qXJjsT_AhUGITQIHbzVCu0Q0pQJegQIDRAB&biw=1904&bih=920&dpr=1#imgrc=HuyGVbW-3jbyMM

Riggio, R. E. (2009, April 18). Pygmalion leadership: The power of positive expectations. *Psychology Today.* Retrieved July 10, 2024, from https://www.psychologytoday.com/us/blog/cutting-edge-leadership/200904/pygmalion-leadership-the-power-of-positive-expectations

Robert Rosenthal. (2009). Social Psychology Network. Retrieved July 10, 2024, from https://rosenthal.socialpsychology.org/

Creditlines

Fig. 13.1: Source: https://panmore.com/pygmalion-effect-and-burnout-when-employees-are-pushed-too-hard.

CHAPTER 14

Edward Locke and Gary Latham's Goal-Setting Theory of Motivation

Do you consider yourself a goal-oriented person? Do you consider yourself more goal oriented than the average person? On a 1 to 10 scale, with 10 being the highest, how would you rate yourself in terms of being goal oriented? Are you more goal oriented in school, your career, or your professional life than in your personal life? Take a moment and reflect on when and how you have gone about setting both personal and professional goals in the past. Are there any tendencies or patterns—either positive or negative—you can identify when you've gone about setting goals? What can you learn from your own experience in goal setting?

College Football Hall of Fame coach Lou Holtz, whose Notre Dame football team went 12–0 and was the consensus national champion in 1988, said that "*if you're bored with life—you don't get up every morning with a burning desire to do things—you don't have enough goals*" (Holtz quoted in Indeed Editorial Team, 2023). Brian Tracy, Canadian-American motivational speaker and bestselling author of over eighty self-development books, said that "*goals are the fuel in the furnace of life. Goals allow you to control the direction of change in your favor. People with clear, written goals, accomplish far more in a shorter period of time than people without them could ever imagine*" (Tracy, 2001).

Setting and achieving goals can provide a sense of purpose, satisfaction, and accomplishment. Moreover, when you set and achieve important, meaningful goals as an individual, as a team, or as an organization, it can make a real difference in your own life and the lives of countless others. American author, poet and philosopher Henry David Thoreau once said:

> *"What you get by achieving your goals is not as important as what you become by achieving your goals."*
>
> (Henry David Thoreau Quotes, 2020)

Background and Overview

Edward Locke found that individuals who set specific, challenging goals performed better than those who set vague, general, easy goals. Those who set goals for themselves, or with others, tend to be more motivated towards achievement and specifically achieving the goals they have set. However, the type and quality of goals an individual sets will affect their level of motivation and how well they will work towards achieving those goals (Mind Tools, n.d.).

Gary Latham studied the effects of goal setting in the workplace, and the results supported Locke's finding:

> There is an inseparable link between goal setting and workplace performance.

Locke and Latham published their seminal work in a book titled *A Theory of Goal Setting & Task Performance* (Locke & Latham, 1990).

Locke and Latham suggested five basic principles of goal setting: clarity, challenge, commitment, feedback, and task complexity.

1. **Clarity**: A clear and measurable goal is more motivational and achievable than one that is vague and nonspecific. Clarity includes a specific target date for achieving the goal.
2. **Challenge**: The goal should be challenging, but not so difficult that it isn't realistic or achievable. A corollary to this is for the goal to be important as well as challenging.
3. **Commitment**: Goal achievement takes commitment on the individual's or the respective team's part. In general, the more important or purposeful the goal, the greater the commitment the

individual or team will likely exhibit towards the goal's achievement. In addition, team commitment is essential when collaboration and teamwork are involved. This is especially important in health care, as the vast majority of work, workflow, and processes require a number of people working efficiently and effectively as a team.

4. **Feedback**: There should be some regular feedback regarding progress being made towards goal achievement. Ongoing monitoring of progress with periodic evaluation should be part of any individual's own process towards goal attainment. Periodic evaluation and feedback can and should include the involvement of team members in a team situation. A key point here is that positive feedback can be encouraging and motivational, while constructive feedback can provide the opportunity for changes or adjustments to be made ongoing, as appropriate.
5. **Task complexity**: The tasks involved with achieving the goal should be challenging, but realistic. Moreover, if the process for completing all the required tasks to achieve the goal are particularly complex, there needs to be ample time for learning, planning, adjustments, and task completion.
(GoStrengths, n.d.)

Locke and Latham's five principles may have been based upon a very similar concept first promulgated in the November 1981 issue of *Management Review* by George Doran, Arthur Miller, and James Cunningham, referred to by the acronym SMART; that is, goals should be specific, measurable, attainable/assignable, realistic, and timely or time specific (Caucci, 2021).

Setting, Monitoring, and Evaluating Goals

Goals help set direction and motivate and drive action. Health care leaders need to become skilled at setting, monitoring, and evaluating goals and their attainment at all levels of the organization. Corporate or organizational goals help establish and convey what the organization believes is most important, as well as help set the overall direction for organizational expectations, effort, and performance. Corporate or organizational goals also provide the structure and important detail for understanding, assessing, and evaluating whether organizational efforts and performance are on track and in line with aspirations, priorities, and expectations.

Goals and objectives at the department, service, or individual employee level must always be in line with, and supportive of, overall organizational mission, vision, priorities, strategy, goals, and objectives. This is referred to as *goal alignment*. It is incumbent on a health care leader—working at any level in the organization—to be sure that department, service, and individual employee goals they are accountable for are in alignment with the organization's mission, vision, strategic direction, priorities, and goals. Moreover, goals and objectives help facilitate the basic management function of control: monitoring progress towards goal achievement and taking any necessary action as needed.

Health care leaders should spend a portion of their time ongoing discussing goals, setting goals, communicating goals, monitoring goals, assessing and evaluating progress towards goal attainment, providing feedback on progress being made towards goal attainment, facilitating action to get back on track towards goal attainment as needed, and recognizing and rewarding workers, as appropriate, for goal attainment. Moreover, while goals help set direction and motivate and drive action, they also facilitate performance appraisal and evaluation.

Improving Customer Experience: An Organizational Goal to Be Cascaded Throughout the Organization

An example of how a goal can help set direction and motivate and drive action using goal alignment is the goal of *improving customer experience* in a hospital. This goal should be specified and promulgated using the SMART goal format (that is, a goal that is written to be specific, measurable, attainable, realistic, and time specific). Therefore, the corporate or organizational goal should be quantified as to the desired performance level. For example, the goal is to achieve the 95th percentage overall for patient satisfaction as measured by the Press Gainy Survey. The department or service-level goal might be to achieve the 95th percentile overall in this department for patient satisfaction as measured by the Press Gainy Survey. Moreover, specific tactics and actions steps can be developed and implemented at the department or service level in pursuit of goal attainment. The individual employee objective (position dependent, of course) might be to consistently provide excellent customer service and achieve a rating of excellent by 95% or more of all patients completing the Press Gainy Survey. Again, specific tactics and action steps can be developed and implemented at the individual employee level in pursuit of goal attainment. This approach helps set direction and motivate and drive action; provides goal alignment; helps facilitate specific tactics and action steps; and helps facilitate performance appraisal and evaluation this is clear, transparent, and objective.

Key Takeaways for Health Care Leaders

Setting goals and objectives can help:

- Clarify and visualize success.
- Clarify purpose, priority, and direction for work performed in the future.
- Add recognizable value to the work employees, leaders, teams, and the organization are doing.
- Provide criteria to monitor and assess progress being made, and to recognize effort and performance towards goal achievement.
- Create tactics for operational or performance efficiencies and improvements as well as time management of tasks and workflow.
- Motivate and increase energy, enthusiasm, effort, and performance in doing the work.
- Enhance teamwork and collaboration.
  (Bard College Center for Civic Engagement, n.d.)

Goals and objectives can and should play an important role in setting expectations for individual and team efforts and performance, as well as facilitate both formal and informal performance evaluation and appraisal. Goal setting can be done for any appropriate time period, including for a calendar year, fiscal year, calendar quarter, month, or an individual employee's performance evaluation or appraisal cycle or time period.

LEADERSHIP ACTION STEPS FOR LOCKE AND LATHAM'S GOAL-SETTING THEORY OF MOTIVATION

1. Start with the end in mind. What does success look like? If we achieve success, how will we know it? How will success be measured? What specific and quantifiable metrics can be used to measure success or achievement of each goal? If working with a group or team, there needs to be ample discussion and consensus regarding what success looks like and how to measure it. Furthermore, don't move past this first step until there is general consensus regarding success and how to define and measure it.
2. Goals should be put in writing and made quantifiable and specific. Written goals are up to 42% more likely to be achieved than goals that aren't written (Tracy, 2004). One study published by Michigan State University Extension, based upon research conducted by Psychology Professor Dr. Gail Matthews, found 76% of those who wrote down their goals and actions, and provided weekly progress updates, successfully achieved their goals, versus only 43% who did not write their goals down (Traugott, 2014).
3. A health care manager's individual goals and objectives should be maintained in a location that is consistently and regularly seen by the health care manager. The same is true for team goals and objectives as well. A regular schedule for assessing progress should be adopted, and with team, departmental, or organizational goals, there should be regular feedback and reporting of the status towards goal achievement. In a team environment, open feedback with discussion regarding the progress being made is important so any necessary adjustments can be made accordingly. Health care worker efforts exhibited and progress made need to be recognized appropriately by health care managers to build positive reinforcement, momentum, and overall motivation. Recognition can also be used as a way to help establish and spur on expectations for future effort and performance. Health care managers need to be sure to provide recognition in concert with equity theory.

4. Large, complex goals should be broken down into smaller, more manageable components or tasks. If the work required to complete a large goal is broken down and components delegated to team members, health care managers should be sure each team member is challenged but not overwhelmed by what they are assigned and provide any necessary training, coaching, and support that team members may require (Mind Tools, n.d.).
5. As a health care manager, use management by objectives when working with subordinates to establish individual employee goals. (See Chapter 11 for more information on this topic.)
6. The management function of control—*monitoring efforts and performance towards goal achievement and taking any necessary corrective action needed* to stay on track towards goal achievement—is absolutely essential throughout this process of setting and working towards achieving goals.

Assessing One's Leadership Style and Locke and Latham's Goal-Setting Theory

The following questions are designed to prompt reflection and self-assessment, and to promote better understanding and insight about how you—as a student, health care manager, or leader—can use or are using Locke and Latham's goal-setting theory of motivation with your own leadership style. Use the following 5-point Likert scale for this assessment:

5 = Always 4 = Sometimes 3 = Neutral 2 = Seldom 1 = Rarely/Never

1. I have individual personal and professional goals that I have committed to writing that are clear, specific, quantifiable, measurable, challenging yet realistic and achievable, and time specific. I keep my individual goals in a location that I can view them, and refer to them regularly.

   5 4 3 2 1

2. I am goal oriented in my role as a health care manager, and work with my subordinates, coworkers, and colleagues to develop important goals and objectives in written SMART goal format that are aligned with overall organizational goals to drive effort, performance, teamwork, collaboration, performance evaluation and appraisal, and overall motivation.

   5 4 3 2 1

3. I break large or complex team or department goals down into smaller, more manageable components. Tasks are delegated to team members in such a way that they are challenged but not overwhelmed, and I provide or arrange to provide any necessary training, coaching, and support needed.

   5 4 3 2 1

4. Written team goals are maintained in a location that can viewed by all members of the team, and referred to by the team, on a regular basis. This includes appropriate status reports detailing progress being made towards goal achievement along with any appropriate recognition.

   5 4 3 2 1

5. I closely monitor the effort and performance of myself and others working towards goal achievement using the basic management function of control. Moreover, I routinely and consistently promote discussion and provide feedback regarding efforts being made towards goal achievement, and appropriately recognize individual and team efforts and performance driving goal achievement to foster motivation.

   5 4 3 2 1

- List two or three of the most frequent ways you do this, and indicate how your subordinates respond to this:
  A.
  B.
  C.

References

Bard College Center for Civic Engagement. (n.d.). *Setting goals and objectives.* Retrieved July 10, 2024, from https://cce.bard.edu/files/Setting-Goals.pdf

Caucci, S. (2021, June 26). Why SMART Goals are Outdated (and Why You Should Leave Them in the Past). 1Huddle. Retrieved July 10, 2024, from https://1huddle.co/blog/outdated-smart-goals/

GoStrengths. (n.d.). *What is goal setting theory?* Retrieved July 10, 2024, from https://gostrengths.com/what-is-goal-setting-theory/

Henry David Thoreau Quotes. (2020, September 26). Spiritual Quotes to Live By. https://spiritualquotestoliveby.com/henry-david-thoreau-quotes/

Indeed Editorial Team. (2023, February 3). *75 quotes about achieving goals to inspire and motivate you. Indeed Career Guide.* Retrieved July 10, 2024, from https://www.indeed.com/career-advice/career-development/achieving-goals-quotes

Locke, E. A., & Latham, G. P. (1990). *A theory of goal setting & task performance.* Prentice Hall.

Mind Tools. (n.d.). *Locke's goal setting theory: Understanding SMART goal setting.* Retrieved July 10, 2024, from https://www.mindtools.com/azazlu3/lockes-goal-setting-theory

Tracy, B. (2001). Eat That Frog!: 21 Great Ways to Stop Procrastinating and Get More Done in Less Time. Berrett-Koehler Publishers.

Tracy, B. (2004). Focal Point: A Proven System to Simplify Your Life, Double Your Productivity, and Achieve All Your Goals. AMACOM.

Traugott, J. (2014, August 26). (n.d.). *Achieving your goals: An evidence-based approach.* Michigan State University Extension. Retrieved July 10, 2024, from https://www.canr.msu.edu/news/achieving_your_goals_an_evidence_based_approach

CHAPTER 15

Clayton Alderfer's ERG Theory of Motivation

There are countless stories of people who became nurses because they wanted to be in the caring profession of nursing and make an impact by helping others: Here is one. Samantha graduated from high school, then attended and graduated a two-year community college, where she received her associate degree in nursing. Samantha had to borrow money to pay for her college and graduated with a significant of amount of debt from her school loans. After graduation Samantha became a nurse in a community hospital, working on the medical/surgical inpatient unit. Samantha worked the night shift and many weekends. The first year or so of her career, Samantha couldn't afford anything more than a small apartment in an area of town that wasn't considered the safest, but it provided shelter and was near her work. Samantha's goals included going back to nursing school to receive her bachelor's degree in nursing sometime within the first five years of her nursing practice, with the help of the hospital's tuition assistance program. However, Samantha knew pursuing her baccalaureate degree in nursing wouldn't be easy financially, as the hospital's tuition reimbursement program would only cover half of her tuition expenses. In addition, Samantha was interested in leadership and wanted to gain enough experience that she could be considered for a nursing management position after obtaining her bachelor's degree, with her ultimate goal of someday becoming a chief nursing officer of a hospital.

What need or needs were driving and motivating Samantha during her first several years as a nurse working on the medical/surgical floor of the hospital? Was she concerned and motivated by the fact she lived in a somewhat unsafe part of town and wanted to improve her living situation as soon as she could afford to do so? Was she motivated more by wanting to earn enough income that she could pay back her education loans in a reasonable time period? Was she more motivated by her passion for serving others as a registered nurse? Or was she more motivated by her goal to become a nurse manager someday and then eventually a chief nursing officer? Under Alderfer's ERG theory of motivation, Samantha's motivations could include all of these goals at the same time. ERG theory suggests that individuals can be motivated by different levels of needs or motivations at the same time, as well as have their motivational priorities change in relation to their sense of progress towards goal achievement and purpose.

Background and Overview

Clayton Alderfer's ERG theory of motivation builds on Maslow's hierarchy of needs and suggests that humans have three primary or core needs: existence, relatedness, and growth (ERG). Alderfer's theory states that these needs may be of different levels of priority for different individuals, and their relative importance for an individual may vary over time.

Existence represents physical and psychological needs or survival needs, which is highlighted by the two bottom levels of the pyramid in Maslow's hierarchy of needs. (Physical needs are labeled safety needs on Maslow's hierarchy.) The next level is relatedness, which includes a sense of belonging, community, and good relationships, including with yourself. This level also includes the need for respect and recognition. This level is represented by the two middle levels of self-esteem and belonging on Maslow's hierarchy. The top level in Alderfer's model is growth, which represents self-development, fulfillment, and a sense of achievement. This top level is labeled self-actualization on Maslow's hierarchy.

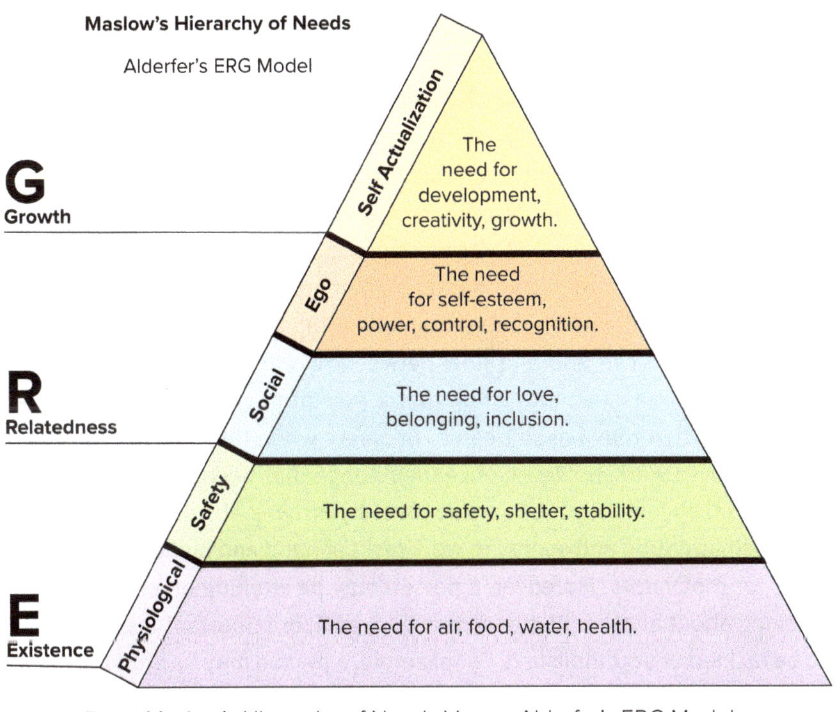

Figure 15.1 Maslow's Hierarchy of Needs Versus Alderfer's ERG Model

This three-factor model of motivation is different from Maslow's hierarchy in that it is fluid, and one doesn't need to have satisfied or substantially satisfied lower-order needs before being motivated by higher-order needs. In the ERG model, one can move between existence, relatedness, and growth levels over time—moving upwards and downwards. Moreover, an individual can be motivated by multiple levels of need at the same time, and the level which is most important to them can change over time as well. The ERG model suggests an individual may prioritize their needs differently than others based upon their own life views. For example, if someone feels they are making great progress in the relatedness need area, even though that need has not been completely or substantially satisfied yet, they may be motivated to pursue the growth need. The opposite of this may be true as well. Someone may feel frustrated in pursuit of their growth need and may even abandon pursuit of this need for a time, while becoming even more motivated to pursue their relatedness need (World of Work, 2019).

The Changing Ebb and Flow of Motivating Factors

In today's world, much credence is given to multitasking. Many of our modern technologies, such as the television, ear buds, computer programs, smartphones, exercise equipment, even cars that steer themselves, provide us with both the incentive and opportunity to multitask. In general, multitasking is viewed as a way for a person to be more productive in their daily life or work.

ERG theory has at its foundation a similar philosophy or belief, in that a person can be motivated by more than one thing at a time. Moreover, a person's motivation can ebb and flow between two or more motivational factors. It seems reasonable to think that a person might be more motivated by hunger when they haven't eaten, or safety when they are traveling on a bus or train to work; however, once their hunger has been satisfied by eating and once they feel they are in a safe place by arriving at work, a person may turn their attention and energy to work tasks at hand and higher-order needs, goals, or motivators. Moreover, a person may be working on one task while thinking about another higher-order need, goal, or important task that is yet to be tackled or accomplished. For example, a person may be drinking or eating while reading a journal article on a pertinent topic that outlines information he or she might incorporate into their work. Moreover, the article might even provide the person with a thought or idea that is highly motivating and inspires the person to strive to achieve a high-level goal or aspiration they have that is in line with their position and organization.

Health care leaders should be cognizant that workers may have more than one factor motivating them at a time, and their motivation level can ebb and flow between more than one motivator as well. Staying connected with workers and understanding each one individually is important for a health care leader to understand how and why a worker may be more or less motivated towards a given task, assignment, or the work at hand at a particular point in time. Realizing that all health care workers have different motivators, a health care leader should work to understand what those motivators are, which ones are more important to the employee, and which one(s) might be in play at any given time. Moreover, different motivators can ebb and flow for an individual. For example, if a health care worker receives an unpleasant telephone call or bad news at work about a family member, their motivators at play in that moment will probably change or at least be reprioritized. And depending on the situation at hand, a health care worker's motivators at play may be changed or reprioritized for a short period of time, or for a much longer period of time.

Key Takeaways for Health Care Leaders

In an article by C. A. Arnolds and Christo Boshoff published in *The International Journal of Human Resource Management*, titled "Compensation, Esteem Valence and Job Performance: An Empirical Assessment of Alderfer's ERG Theory," the authors cite empirical research showing "that esteem as a personality variable exerts a significant influence on the job performance of both top managers and frontline employees" (Arnolds & Boshoff, 2002). This suggests that a health care manager must really understand that a subordinate has various needs—not just one—that must be satisfied at the same time. If the health care worker feels they aren't being provided with opportunities for growth and advancement, they may become frustrated and be much more motivated to pursue their need for relatedness. As a result, the health care worker may begin spending an excessive amount of time socializing at work, until they feel the organizational environment, employment situation, or even the manager's leadership style and management of them as a subordinate, will provide the employee with growth and advancement opportunities (Management Study Guide, n.d.).

Health care managers must expect the needs of their subordinates and teams to change over time, and even to ebb and flow between the three needs of growth, relatedness, and existence. Moreover, health care leaders must know and understand each of their subordinates' needs and how they prioritize those needs at any given point in time. In this way, a health care manager can alter their approach with an individual health care worker based upon the most dominant and pressing needs of the subordinate, while not overlooking other needs that are important at the same time. As mentioned in other chapters in this handbook, the concept of situational leadership—managing each employee differently based upon their job readiness and psychological readiness at any point in time—applies here with Alderfer's ERG theory of motivation.

LEADERSHIP ACTION STEPS FOR ALDERFER'S ERG THEORY OF MOTIVATION

1. Health care managers should create an environment where the basic, lower-order needs of health care workers are continually and consistently being met. This includes creating a working environment where health care workers feel safe and secure and are provided with the appropriate resources, including personal protective equipment and related infection control policies and procedures that protect them from infections and contagious diseases that can be transmitted from patients and others. This also includes providing for basic existence needs, such as access to clean drinking water, coffee, snacks, and other refreshments at break times, with access to appropriate areas where they can eat and take breaks from the demands of their work. Occasional surprise refreshments for health care workers go a long way to not only help meet physiological needs, but also the need for belongingness, appreciation, and respect. In addition, existence needs of health care workers include basic training to help them avoid contracting infections and other contagious diseases from patients. These steps will appeal to the health care worker's need for existence.
2. Health care managers should make sure subordinates' work schedules accurately reflect the appropriate days/shifts/times they are to work, and that worker compensation is accurate and reflects all hours worked, as well as nonproductive hours that should be paid. These steps will appeal to the health care worker's need for existence.
3. Health care managers should create an open environment where all health care workers can speak their mind and offer their opinion and suggestions without fear of personal judgment, ridicule, condemnation, or reprisal. Moreover, health care managers should promote an atmosphere where employees feel appreciated, cared for, and part of the team that is doing something of the highest importance together: caring for and serving patients in their time of need. These steps will appeal to the health care worker's need for relatedness.
4. Health care managers should always be honest and trustworthy. Health care managers need to be good listeners and empower their subordinates by providing them with as much freedom and autonomy

as possible, allowing them to use their creativity to help problem-solve and improve individual and organizational efficiency and performance. Moreover, health care managers should provide positive, appropriate, and timely feedback to subordinates as it relates to the care they are providing or service they are rendering, and the difference it is making in the lives of patients and families being served. These steps will appeal to the health care worker's need for relatedness and growth.

5. Health care managers need to make sure every subordinate is involved and engaged in their work and clearly see and understand how their work impacts and contributes to the team, as well as to others in the organization, including patients and families. These steps will appeal to the health care worker's need for relatedness and growth.
6. Health care managers should recognize the good work their employees and teams are doing, and clearly highlight how that work contributes to quality patient care, patient experience and satisfaction, teamwork, and the pursuit of organizational goals, mission, and vision. Moreover, health care managers should provide regular feedback to subordinates, as well as periodically express how the employee contributes to and is a vital part of the health care team that is positively impacting lives and the community being served. Building a spirit of teamwork and collaboration is also important and can include company culture training and company-sponsored functions that bring employees and teams together. These steps will appeal to the health care worker's need for relatedness and growth.
7. Health care managers should get to know and understand each subordinate and their goals, potential, and performance capabilities, and look for opportunities, tasks, and projects where the employee can work towards achieving important work and career objectives, demonstrating their individual potential as well as ability to significantly contribute to the team and the organization. Employee training, career coaching, mentoring, creative and challenging projects and assignments, and leadership inspiration to move beyond the employee's comfort zone can all help the employee to feel empowered and move his efforts and contributions closer to his highest potential. These steps will appeal to the health care worker's need for growth.

Assessing One's Leadership Style and Alderfer's ERG Theory of Motivation

The following questions are designed to prompt reflection and self-assessment, and to promote better understanding and insight about how you—as a student, health care manager, or leader—can use or are using Alderfer's ERG theory of motivation with your own leadership style. Use the following 5-point Likert scale for this assessment:

5 = Always 4 = Sometimes 3 = Neutral 2 = Seldom 1 = Rarely/Never

1. I routinely and consistently work to make sure my subordinates' basic needs of safety and security are being met in their working environment, and that they have all the necessary training, coaching, and resources to keep themselves, their coworkers, and their patients safe.

   5 4 3 2 1

2. I routinely and consistently work to make sure my subordinates' basic needs for coffee, tea, soda, cold drinking water, snacks, and refreshments are met, along with having an appropriate break area to help foster camaraderie. Moreover, I work to make sure my subordinates always get their needed breaks and lunch period away from the demands of work and recognize the importance of same.

   5 4 3 2 1

3. I routinely and consistently keep my promises, don't make promises I can't keep, and respectfully tell the truth, which my subordinates can always count on.

   5 4 3 2 1

4. I routinely and consistently provide my subordinates and teams with as much freedom and autonomy in their work as possible, making sure they have clear direction, support, and understanding of my expectations for their effort and performance.

5 4 3 2 1

5. I routinely and consistently solicit suggestions and ideas from my subordinates and teams and utilize and implement as many of them as possible, providing positive feedback and recognition for their efforts and contributions and the impact they are making.

5 4 3 2 1

- List two or three of the most frequent ways you do this, and indicate how your subordinates typically react:
  A.
  B.
  C.

6. I get to know and fully understand my subordinates and their values, goals, needs, and desires regarding their work and the working environment; provide them with support, coaching, and mentoring as needed; and provide them with as many opportunities as possible to demonstrate their performance capabilities while recognizing same with regular feedback.

5 4 3 2 1

____

____

____

____

References

Arnolds, C. A., & Boshoff, C. (2002). Compensation, esteem valence and job performance: An empirical assessment of Alderfer's ERG theory. *The International Journal of Human Resource Management, 13*(4), 697–719. https://doi.org/10.1080/09585190210125868

Management Study Guide. (n.d.). *ERG theory of motivation.* Retrieved July 10, 2024, from https://www.managementstudyguide.com/erg-theory-motivation.htm

World of Work. (2019, February). *Alderfer's ERG theory of motivation: A simple summary.* Retrieved July 10, 2024, from https://worldofwork.io/2019/02/alderfers-erg-theory-of-motivation/

Creditlines

Fig. 15.1: Source: https://worldofwork.io/2019/02/alderfers-erg-theory-of-motivation/.

Fig. 15.1a: Copyright © 2019 Depositphotos/ShadeDesign.sd.

CHAPTER 16

Julian Rappaport's Empowerment Theory of Motivation

Have you ever worked for a boss who was empowering: a boss who provided you with freedom, autonomy, control, and decision-making authority regarding your work, work assignments, work tasks, work processes, and other decisions affecting the elements of the work environment? Conversely, have you ever worked for a boss who was a micromanager—a boss with a directive style of management, who was controlling, provided you with little to no autonomy and freedom, gave highly specific instructions about how to do tasks and assignments, and made most all the decisions regarding your work and the work environment? What a stark contrast in leadership styles between a boss who is empowering and a boss who is a controlling micromanager! The vast majority of us much prefer to work for a boss who is empowering, and not a controlling micromanager. When employees feel empowered, they are typically more productive, more creative, more effective, more motivated, and genuinely more satisfied with their boss, their work, and their organization.

Background and Overview

Julian Rappaport is an American psychologist who first introduced the concept of empowerment in social work and social psychiatry. At the time of this writing, Rappaport is professor emeritus at the University of Illinois at Urbana-Champaign in Urbana, Illinois. Working in the field of community psychology and social psychiatry, Rappaport's seminal work on empowerment resulted in his 1984 book *Studies in Empowerment* (Rappaport, 1984).

The concept of empowerment in leadership concerns the process of giving frontline employees the authority to make decisions that were once reserved only for managers (LaMarco, 2018). Empowerment is about authority being delegated to employees that provides them with a level of freedom, autonomy, control, and decision-making authority regarding their work, work processes, and working environment. Furthermore, empowerment is not necessarily reserved for frontline employees, but can also include virtually anyone, such as caregivers, health care workers, and frontline and middle managers. Empowerment is the process of a health care manager—at any level—allowing more freedom, more autonomy, more control, and more decision-making authority to a subordinate, health care worker, or team. Empowerment is the opposite of a more traditional or historical management style that includes command and control; that is, a management style that is directive, controlling, and authoritarian, and where managers maintain most all of the power, authority, and control in the organization. The command-and-control style of management was common during the industrial revolution and even throughout the middle part of the 20th century, when tasks and assignments were assigned to employees who had little to no input regarding the assignments, tasks, or how best to carry those assignments or tasks out—a Theory X concept of leadership, if you will. Empowerment, on the other hand, is a style of leadership that supports the Theory Y belief and style. (See Chapter 8 for more information on the topic.)

Empowerment Can Be Positive for Both Health Care Leaders and Workers Alike

When done appropriately, empowerment can be positive for both health care leaders and workers alike. For example, most health care workers who have experience and have worked in their organization for some time seek empowerment from their health care leader. They desire freedom and autonomy to do their work, authority to make decisions concerning their work, and support and encouragement from their health care leaders. When health care leaders empower their workers, they are also making a positive impact on employee motivation, morale, commitment, loyalty, satisfaction, and the overall employment relationship. However, there is more to this story.

Health care leaders who empower their workers are actually providing themselves with more time to focus on other important tasks and responsibilities with their leadership role. How? As discussed, the opposite of empowerment is micromanagement, and micromanagement typically takes more of a leader's time and effort. Health care leaders who are overly controlling, provide more direction and instructions than needed, make all the decisions or the vast majority of them, and closely supervise employees, are spending more time unnecessarily on these things. As a result, health care leaders who empower their employees tend to foster creativity, innovation, and problem-solving along with all the other positive attributes of empowerment previously noted, including saving the leader time and effort. Moreover, health care leaders who are empowering are helping to reduce health care worker burnout, while promoting employee recruitment and retention as well as productivity.

Key Takeaways for Health Care Leaders

Without the trust of subordinates, colleagues, and coworkers, a health care manager will not be effective. A health care manager must be trustworthy in order to have credibility and believability, and trust is built with authenticity. Without trust and authenticity, health care workers will be skeptical of whatever the health care manager does and says. For example, if the health care manager provides autonomy, freedom, and control to the subordinate or team to complete an assignment or task, will the subordinate's or team's decisions or work methods be second-guessed by the health care manager? If the health care manager delegates a level of decision-making authority to the subordinate or team, will the health care manager support the decision? If there are real questions about the health care manager's commitment, follow-through, trust, or support when providing or delegating freedom, autonomy, control, and decision-making to a subordinate or team, will the subordinate or team give their best effort or performance if they don't believe in their boss's word? Therefore, trustworthiness is absolutely essential for any health care manager to possess in order to empower subordinates and others.

Health care managers must also be cognizant of providing employees all the information, resources, and authority needed to complete the work they've been empowered to do. As Julian Rappaport famously stated:

> *"Having rights but no resources and no services available is a cruel joke."*
>
> (Rappaport, 1981).

When a health care manager is providing subordinates or teams with autonomy, freedom, control, and decision-making authority, he must be clear regarding the goals and objectives to be accomplished. Subordinates and teams must fully understand the goals and objectives, along with their purpose—the *why*—in order to create and appropriately shape their approach, methods, and decisions relating to assignments and tasks they are to pursue; and the work, work process, and work flow they are doing and producing independently and collectively—to be the most effective when empowered. Understanding the *why* helps employees better understand *how* to complete tasks most efficiently and effectively to achieve the goals and objectives at hand.

LEADERSHIP ACTION STEPS FOR EMPOWERMENT

An article by Susan M. Heathfield (2020) titled "*Top 10 Principles of Employee Empowerment*" lists the following 10 action steps for leaders to use to empower employees:

1. **Demonstrate that you value people**—by what you say, what you do, how you talk, and your body language.
2. **Share leadership vision**—and use participatory leadership in the process.
3. **Share goals and direction**—again, using participatory leadership in the process.
4. **Trust people**—and set clear expectations and agree upon what success looks like.
5. **Provide needed information for decision-making**—being sure your employees have all the information and resources needed to complete tasks and goals successfully.
6. **Delegate authority with impact opportunities**—that are meaningful, not just more work.
7. **Provide frequent feedback**—both positive and constructive feedback, making the most of opportunities to coach, guide, and foster employee development.
8. **Focus on solving problems**—and avoid finger-pointing and blaming.

9. **Ask questions, listen, and learn**—using appropriately probing questions to solve problems, promote understanding, and guide learning and development.
10. **Recognize and reward empowered behavior**—so that employees feel appreciated and valued. Moreover, it is through recognition and reward of empowered behavior that employees will put forth more of their discretionary effort: that is, effort and performance above and beyond the minimum requirements or acceptable standards.

Assessing One's Leadership Style and Rappaport's Empowerment Theory of Motivation

The following questions are designed to prompt reflection and self-assessment, and to promote better understanding and insight about how you—as a student, health care manager, or leader—can use or are using Rappaport's empowerment theory of motivation with subordinates and teams using your own leadership style. Use the following 5-point Likert scale for this assessment:

5 = Always 4 = Sometimes 3 = Neutral 2 = Seldom 1 = Rarely/Never

1. I routinely and consistently display my trust in subordinates and teams by providing them with autonomy, freedom, control, and authority to make decisions that significantly impact their work, important organizational goals, and the working environment.

   5 4 3 2 1

2. I routinely and consistently communicate the mission and vision of the organization and department, use participatory leadership in establishing goals and objectives, and provide subordinates and teams with clear information and support to accomplish tasks and goals.

   5 4 3 2 1

3. I routinely and consistently ask questions and listen, provide subordinates and teams with positive and constructive feedback as appropriate, and provide coaching and advising as appropriate for purposes of facilitating learning, understanding, growth, and development.

5 4 3 2 1

4. I routinely and consistently focus on solving problems and improving performance and create an environment where subordinates and teams do the same, while avoiding finger-pointing and blame.

5 4 3 2 1

5. I routinely and consistently acknowledge, recognize, and reward subordinates and teams as appropriate when empowered for their efforts, work, and performance.

5 4 3 2 1

- List two or three of the ways you do this:
  A.
  B.
  C.

____

____

____

____

References

Heathfield, S. M. (2020, April 3). Top 10 principles of employee empowerment. liveaboutdotcom. https://www.liveabout.com/top-principles-of-employee-empowerment-1918658

LaMarco, N. (2018, December 3). *The concept of empowerment in leadership. Chron.* Retrieved July 10, 2024, from https://smallbusiness.chron.com/concept-empowerment-leadership-15371.html

Rappaport, J. (1981). "In praise of paradox. A social policy of empowerment over prevention" (PDF). *American Journal of Community Psychology, 9*(1): 1–25 (13). doi:10.1007/BF00896357.

Rappaport, J. (1984). *Studies in empowerment: Steps toward understanding and action.* Haworth Press.

CHAPTER 17

Concluding Remarks

The financing and delivery of health care in the United States has changed dramatically over time. Once thought of as a cottage industry, much of the inpatient care during the early 20th century was provided in private, physician-owned homes that had been converted to hospitals, or in public hospitals which weren't much more than sanitariums. Hospital and health care services were paid for out of pocket, as commercial health insurance didn't come on the scene until sometime in the 1930s, and Medicare and Medicaid didn't exist until 1966.

Prior to the publication of the Flexner Report in 1910, medical education and training was still fairly primitive and suffered from a lack of standards or even requirements, such as postgraduate or residency training. In the early 1900s, many physicians were local practitioners whose exclusive medical training was through an apprenticeship (Ludmerer, 2010). Today, medical education is a postgraduate endeavor that takes four years. After graduation from medical school, a physician then enters into a residency program in the specialty of choice, which is typically a minimum of three years in duration. Physicians wanting to specialize in a subspecialty of medicine, such as orthopedic spine surgery, musculoskeletal MRI radiology, or cancer surgery, might complete a postresidency fellowship of one or more additional years. And today's medical education and training are based upon modern standards, requirements, research, and evidence-based medicine; all a far cry from the early 1900s, when the X-ray and even penicillin hadn't been discovered.

Today so much has changed, and continues to change, in health care: Drugs, chemotherapy agents, diagnostic equipment, surgical instruments, anesthesia, the use of advanced technologies and computer systems, the environment of care, and even the way health care is reimbursed have all changed dramatically. Changes in these and other areas will most certainly continue as health care evolves.

Today's modern hospital is one of the more complex organizations there is, and the efficient and effective management of hospitals is increasingly becoming more challenging as expectations in all stakeholder segments increase. However, it can be said that the clinical capabilities, the clinical care, and the clinical outcomes provided by U.S. hospitals—as well as other health service organizations delivering direct patient care today—are nothing less than amazing. Many of the interventions and clinical procedures being done routinely today in hospitals, diagnostic centers, ambulatory surgery centers, outpatient clinics, and even physician offices were unheard of just a few short decades ago. Much of what was once considered care and treatment that could only be provided on an inpatient basis is being done today on an outpatient basis. Yes, the cost of health care continues to increase at a fast pace which some maintain isn't sustainable. Yet our clinical capabilities, clinical quality, clinical safety, patient experience, and patient outcomes have never been better.

From my experience, the vast majority of health care workers go into the health care field to make an impact—a difference in the lives of others. As a hospital administrator, most health care workers that I've known or worked with, or even interacted with or been cared for as a patient myself, have been dedicated, caring people committed to helping others. For most, working in health care is a calling to service. The provision of health care services still remains a noble profession today, with caregivers held in high regard. Most patients and families in the United States are extremely grateful and thankful for those caregivers who serve them and care for them in their time of need. But what can be an extraordinary experience in a hospital for a patient can be just an ordinary day for a caregiver. And while providing care and service to patients can be an extremely rewarding and gratifying experience for the caregiver, it isn't void of its own unique demands and challenges either.

A growing challenge for virtually all health care organizations and leaders is the problem of manpower shortages and burnout. Hospitals as well as other health care organizations are experiencing shortages in manpower in almost every area, department, and discipline. While this is a national—maybe even international—problem, it is compounded by a heightening of burnout being experienced by most every discipline in a hospital, including physicians, nurses, technicians, therapists, and others. An article by the American Medical Association (AMA) states that "physician burnout is a long-term stress reaction which can include emotional exhaustion, depersonalization or lack of empathy, and a feeling of decreased personal achievement. Burnout is a condition that affects all specialties and all practice settings. Physician burnout is an epidemic in the U.S. health care system, with nearly 63% of physicians reporting signs of burnout" (American Medical Association, 2023). In the article, Christine Sinsky, MD, AMA vice president of professional satisfaction, states that "while burnout manifests in individuals, it originates in systems. Burnout is not the result of a deficiency in resiliency among physicians, rather it is due to the systems in which physicians work." Physician burnout reduces their productivity and morale, which can also lead to a reduction in the quality and time spent in delivering patient care. And physician burnout is on the rise. Like most other problems and challenges health care leaders must confront, burnout is one that is multifaceted and complex. Nonetheless, it is a problem and challenge that many health care leaders must face head-on, and be motivated to do so.

In an era when all health care stakeholders are expecting more and even demanding more from their hospitals, health care service organizations, and providers, health care leaders who are motivating and inspiring are needed now—and for the foreseeable future—more than ever. The fundamental principles and techniques learned and applied from the motivational theories highlighted in this book can make an impact and a difference in countless lives, including both those providing health care and those receiving health care. For health care leaders who want to make a real difference in health care and the word at large, becoming a genuine, authentic, effective motivator of others can help make the leader's calling to make a difference with service above self a reality.

In thinking about the informal and formal leaders who have made a real difference in my life, I can't help but think about their encouragement, support, attention, feedback, reinforcement, and belief in me that motivated and empowered me to set important goals, work hard to achieve them, and work towards my highest level of potential. Their motivation still encourages me today and drives me towards self-actualization, reaching my highest level of potential.

Will you become a health care leader who can be all you can be, achieve all you can achieve, and help others do the same, with motivation that is inspiring and empowering? Why not you?

References

American Medical Association. (2023, February 16). *What is physician burnout?* Retrieved July 10, 2024, from https://www.ama-assn.org/practice-management/physician-health/what-physician-burnout

Ludmerer, K. M. (2010). Commentary: Understanding the Flexner Report. *Academic Medicine*, *85*(2), 193–196. https://doi.org/10.1097/acm.0b013e3181c8f1e7

Appendix

Applying Motivational Theory in Health Care Leadership: Quick Reference Table

MOTIVATIONAL THEORY	HEALTH CARE MANAGERS SHOULD ...
Charles Darwin and Sigmund Freud's instinct theory	• Be self-aware of their own basic life instincts and how these instincts drive or motivate them in leadership and everyday life. • Listen to their own intuition for people, problems, and situations and how it can be applied using *emotional intelligence (EI)*. • Constantly be aware of their own ego/personality and how it shapes and directs their thoughts, actions, and leadership. • Get to know their employees on a personal level and understand the basic life instincts that motivate them.

MOTIVATIONAL THEORY	HEALTH CARE MANAGERS SHOULD ...
Edward Lee Thorndike's feedback intervention theory	• Ask employees about their preferences for feedback and honor such preferences. • Provide authentic, honest feedback to employees based upon the manager's first-hand knowledge and observations. • Provide positive feedback in a private or public setting as appropriate, but constructive/negative feedback in private. • Use the concept of *situational leadership* and *emotional intelligence* to be effective and appropriate with feedback, including mediums/ channels and frequency.
Abraham Maslow's hierarchy of needs theory	• Ask employees about their needs and understand the importance of each to the employee. • Expect employee needs to change over time. • Consistently and continually satisfy lower-order employee needs. • Create opportunities where employees feel empowered and can pursue higher-order needs in their work to help bring them intrinsic satisfaction and fulfillment.

MOTIVATIONAL THEORY	HEALTH CARE MANAGERS SHOULD ...
B.F. Skinner's reinforcement theory	• Provide positive and negative reinforcement that is appropriate given the situation/employee's effort and performance. • Be cognizant about the way positive or negative reinforcement is carried out or delivered; this is more important than the amount. • Be authentic and follow through with any reinforcement efforts that have been hinted at or suggested to the employee. • Understand employees will use *equity theory* to compare the type and frequency of feedback and reinforcement they receive to that which other employees receive.
Frederick Herzberg's two-factor/ hygiene theory	• Understand that hygiene factors such as compensation, status, and working environment don't motivate employees or promote job satisfaction; however, the inadequacy of hygiene factors can create job dissatisfaction. • Certain hygiene factors require constant reinforcement to not be perceived or experienced as demotivators. • Motivating factors are job content factors, or those things which are intrinsic to the work itself, such as growth opportunities, empowerment, and satisfaction provided by the work. • Job enrichment is a central method to engendering greater employee motivation, including greater effort and performance.

MOTIVATIONAL THEORY	HEALTH CARE MANAGERS SHOULD ...
The Hawthorne effect	• Acknowledge, recognize, and pay attention to employees. • Observe employees performing tasks and doing work in their work areas. • Show appreciation and respect to employees for their efforts, performance, and contributions. • Treat employees like volunteers who can leave the organization anytime they want. • Use *management by walking around* frequently to be visible, observe, and interact with employees.
Douglas McGregor's Theory X and Theory Y	• Be self-aware and understand their own predisposition or belief towards whether most employees will be responsible, work hard, and can be trusted, or are lazy and must be closely supervised at all times. • Listen to employee language, observe attitudes and behaviors, and monitor employee effort and performance to understand each employee's job readiness and psychological readiness. • Understand how to apply *situational leadership theory*—a mixture of *Theory X and Theory Y* approaches—depending upon the employee's psychological and job readiness. • Be cognizant of today's societal and cultural norms that favor a *Theory Y* leadership style. However, at the same time understand the organizational culture and how it impacts the amount of freedom and autonomy that can be provided to employees.

MOTIVATIONAL THEORY	HEALTH CARE MANAGERS SHOULD ...
John Stacey Adam's equity theory	• Understand that employees highly value fairness and equity in their treatment/employment relationship and will look at many things regarding how their own treatment compares to others. • Recognize and understand each employee's career goals, as well as overall psychological characteristics and generally what each one considers important in their employment relationship. • Always be fair, equitable, and consistent in the treatment of employees. • Use a high degree of e*motional intelligence (EI*) in monitoring and assessing how employees are perceiving their treatment in terms of it being fair and equitable.
Victor H. Vroom's expectancy theory	• Know and understand employee capabilities, wants, and desires in order to properly connect employee effort and performance to recognition and reward. • Recognize that past precedent for employee recognition and reward creates employee expectations for future recognition and reward. • Be sure employee recognition and reward aligns with company goals, policies, and organizational culture. • Understand that employees will assess how the recognition and reward provided to others compares with their own (see *equity theory*).

MOTIVATIONAL THEORY	HEALTH CARE MANAGERS SHOULD ...
Peter Drucker's management by objectives (MBO)	• Use *participatory leadership* in carrying out the *MBO* process, thus making it collaborative and supportive. • Be well trained in how to collaboratively apply *MBO* and make sure there is complete goal alignment with employee, departmental, and organizational goals. • Make sure that individual employee objectives are written to be specific, measurable, achievable, realistic and timely/time specific (*SMART* format). • Lead by example with their own written goals, using transparency with goals, and model the way for employees to follow.
Fred Edward Fiedler's contingency theory	• Be self-aware and understand their own natural leadership style, and how this style can be used most effectively to maximize performance in their current leadership position. • Develop strong *emotional intelligence (EI)* over their career to understand their own natural leadership tendencies in different environments and situations. • Be cognizant at all times of both when and how to flex their natural leadership style as needed to best apply *situational leadership*. • Use self-reflection, 360-degree evaluation, and other appropriate methods to identify their own leadership attributes that may need to be developed or enhanced to be a more effective leader, along with a plan to develop same.

MOTIVATIONAL THEORY	HEALTH CARE MANAGERS SHOULD ...
Robert Rosenthal's Pygmalion theory	• Clearly understand the performance capabilities of their employees, as well as the employee's own expectations. • Make sure expectations established for self and others are clear, realistic, well known and understood, as well as high but achievable and appropriate. • Outwardly demonstrate trust, confidence, belief, and support in employees consistently. • Provide positive feedback and reinforce expectations and beliefs about goals and accomplishments that have been achieved, as well as those that can be achieved in the future.
Edwin A. Locke's goal-setting theory	• Use *MBO* at the employee level, and make sure there is goal alignment between organizational goals, departmental goals, and individual employee goals. • Put goals in the *SMART* format so they are specific, measurable, attainable, realistic, and time specific. • Put goals in writing and keep them where they will be read and referred to frequently. • Monitor progress towards goal achievement ongoing, and provide appropriate feedback, communication, and reporting regarding progress being made, using goals as one factor in employee appraisal.

MOTIVATIONAL THEORY	HEALTH CARE MANAGERS SHOULD ...
Clayton Alderfer's ERG theory	• Expect employee needs to change over time, and ebb and flow between the three needs of growth, relatedness, and existence. • Create an environment where basic, lower-order needs of employees are continually and consistently being met. • Create an open environment where all employees feel welcome, can openly speak their mind, and feel a strong sense of camaraderie and team. • Know and understand each employee and their goals and capabilities; look for opportunities where the employee can work towards achieving their career goals and potential.
Julian Rappaport's empowerment theory	• Be authentic, honest, and trustworthy at all times, remembering that employees volunteer their discretionary effort (the extra effort they have to give). • Delegate decisions, tasks, and projects from the beginning, allowing employees freedom to innovate and do the work as they deem most appropriate. • Accept that not all employee-made decisions will turn out exactly as desired; however, hold employees accountable for results while being supportive and understanding. • Look for coachable/teachable moments and opportunities to use employee experiences to help them grow, learn, and develop.

Source: Reed, S. B. (2019). Becoming a Healthcare Leader (Second Edition). Cognella.

Glossary

The following selected terms and definitions are used in this handbook. Use this listing as a reference, as needed, when you encounter one of these terms.

Discretionary effort—the effort an individual employee is giving, or willing to give, at any time above and beyond the minimum acceptable or expected standards or requirements (Reed, 2019).

Emotional intelligence—the ability to be self-aware, understand and manage your own emotions as well as perceive and understand the emotions of those around you (www.wikipedia.com).

Employee—an individual who is employed by, and working for, an organization at any given level in the organizational structure (Reed, 2019).

Empowerment—delegating management authority and autonomy to others, providing them control, problem-solving, creative thinking and decision-making (Reed, 2019).

Health care leader—also referred to as a leader, this is a manager who is in a position of authority and responsibility in a hospital's or health service organization's chain of command. This can be a health care manager position from a frontline supervisor to the chief executive officer.

Health care manager—a position of authority and responsibility in a hospital's or health service organization's chain of command, typically with responsibility for supervising one or more health care workers.

Health care worker—an employee working in a hospital or other health service organization in any position, full time or part time, whether in a direct patient care role or support service role.

Leadership—motivating and inspiring others to work hard to achieve organizational goals (Reed, 2019).

Leadership motivation—motivation and inspiration provided by a health care manager to one or more health care workers or teams.

Management—the process of coordinating, organizing, and supervising the people and tasks of a company or group in order to achieve the company or group's goals. Getting work done through others (Reed, 2019).

Motivation—the set of forces that initiates, directs, and makes people persist in their efforts to accomplish a goal (Reed, 2019).

Participatory leadership—a style of leadership in which the leader encourages, supports, solicits, and values employee input in decision-making (Reed, 2019).

Senior leadership—health care managers who hold executive leadership positions at the top of a company's organizational chart or chain of command, typically having management responsibility that is broad in scope (Reed, 2019).

Servant leadership—a style of leadership in which leaders focus on serving those around them, sharing power, and facilitating others' work, rather than accumulating power for themselves and wielding that power by directing others (Reed, 2019).

Situational leadership—an approach to leadership in which the leader adjusts his or her style to the particular needs of the followers, placing importance on subordinate's job readiness (knowledge, skills, ability, and experience to do the job) and psychological readiness (motivation and willingness to do the job) (Reed, 2019).

Subordinate—an employee or health care worker who reports to a manager (supervisor) who typically holds a higher position of greater authority in the organization's hierarchy or chain of command.

Supervisor—a health care manager who is administratively responsible for one or more health care workers (subordinates). This includes health care managers who supervise another health care manager and hold a higher position of greater authority in the organization's hierarchy or chain of command.

Transformational leadership—(a) a leadership style and outcome based on leaders working with employees and teams to identify needed change, creating a vision to guide the change through inspiration, and executing the change in tandem with highly committed employees; and (b) a leadership style that transforms an organization and its people into high performers (Reed, 2019).

References

Reed, S. B. (2019). Becoming a Healthcare Leader (Second Edition). Cognella.

Index

A

B

C

L

M

N

O

P

R

S

T

U

V

W

X

www.ingramcontent.com/pod-product-compliance
Ingram Content Group UK Ltd.
Pitfield, Milton Keynes, MK11 3LW, UK
UKHW021830270726
14058UKWH00001B/77

9 798823 327299